Quantum
Wellness

Quantum
Wellness

Kathy Freston

LONDON

1 3 5 7 9 10 8 6 4 2

This edition published in 2008 by Vermilion, an imprint of Ebury Publishing

Ebury Publishing is a Random House Group company

Originally published in 2008 in the United States by Weinstein Books

The Random House Group Limited Reg. No. 954009

Addresses for companies within the Random House Group can be found at
www.rbooks.co.uk

A CIP catalogue record for this book is available from the British Library

The Random House Group Limited supports The Forest Stewardship
Council (FSC), the leading international forest certification organisation.
All our titles that are printed on Greenpeace approved FSC certified paper
carry the FSC logo. Our paper procurement policy can be found at
www.rbooks.co.uk/environment

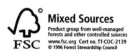

Mixed Sources
Product group from well-managed
forests and other controlled sources
www.fsc.org Cert no. TT-COC-2139
© 1996 Forest Stewardship Council

Printed and bound by Griffin Press in Australia and
in the UK by CPI Mackays, Chatham ME5 8TD

ISBN 978 0 09 192915 2

Copies are available at special rates for bulk orders. Contact the sales development
team on 020 7840 8487 for more information.

To buy books by your favourite authors and register for offers, visit www.rbooks.co.uk

For Tom

CONTENTS

Contents

ACKNOWLEDGMENTS

WHEN HARVEY WEINSTEIN FIRST SUGGESTED THAT I WRITE A BOOK ON wellness, I thought, "Who am I to speak on such a broad and complex subject?" But respecting Harvey's instincts as I do, I began to take seriously the ideas and pieces of the puzzle that had been working their way into my awareness for some time. He was right (as is usually the case) in that there was a hunger for a new approach to feeling good and healing on multiple levels. So thank you to Harvey for the big idea.

And to Rob Weisbach, who took the big idea and honed it into a workable thesis of "small steps, huge results." He stayed with me as I developed the book, herding my thoughts and ideas into a consistent message. He and the team at Weinstein Books—Judy Hottensen, Katie Finch, Camille March, Kristin Powers, Emily Wilkinson, Adrian Palacios, and Richard Florest—are among the most creative, savvy, and passionate people I've ever had the honor to work with.

I am so very privileged to have a Foreword by the brilliant Dr. Mehmet Oz, who strikes that incredible balance of progressive thinking and academic knowledge. Lisa Oz is always adding in the alternative spiritual juice that I love. I am fortified by their friendship and I thank them both. I'm also deeply thankful to know and learn from

Dr. Andrew Weil, Dr. Neal Barnard, Dr. Dean Ornish, Dr. Drew Francis, and Dr. Soram Singh Khalsa. And my friend Marianne Williamson was a teacher to me before I ever met her. I am always humbled and in awe of her illuminations.

A huge and heartfelt thanks to my editor, Caroline Pincus, without whom I could not have birthed this baby. She often said things better than I could have and in ways that were almost magical. It has been such a joy to work with someone who is so talented and skillful, so astute at distilling and alchemizing the words so that the message would be clear.

I have so much appreciation for Jennifer Rudolph Walsh, Jim Wiatt, and my home at William Morris; I count my lucky stars to have their expert guidance and enthusiasm.

And there is my ongoing gratitude toward those who have opened my eyes to the issues of vegetarianism. At the top of the list is Bruce Friedrich, who is tireless and selfless in his mission to educate people about the truth of what happens to animals behind closed doors. He has helped me to articulate what I think is an emerging shift in consciousness about food and human decency. Jannette Patterson and Lisa Lange have kept me well informed, gently pulling me past my comfort levels so that I would continue to upgrade my values and ethics. My thanks go to Tal Ronnen, an inspired chef. He helps make becoming vegan a delicious and easy endeavor.

Olivia Rosewood, a brilliant researcher and writer herself, put together so much information for this book that is both prudent and insightful; I could not have done this without her.

To Nicki Graham, who has been ever present with anything and everything that was needed to complete this project, I am grateful. And Brian Nice, the incredible photographer, thank you!

Finally, the last couple of years have been ones of extreme

growth and awakening for me. Thank you to the teachers I've been lucky enough to work with: Armand Bytton, Barry Michels, Christine Price. I am so lifted by the insight and wisdom that I have received from each of them.

FOREWORD

THIS IS NOT A TYPICAL HEALTH BOOK. NO MAGIC FOODS OR PILLS OR miracle procedures are offered here. No, the medicine prescribed by Kathy Freston is something much more potent. As a heart surgeon, I frequently see people who are not carrying a "disease" but who are also not well. They are not thriving the way we all desire. In fact, a diagnosis of disease, which is usually doled out by well-meaning physicians desiring to satisfy the curiosity of patients who have finally sought their help, probably explains only a fraction of the lack of health felt by many people. Why? Because real wellness is much more than the lack of disease. Health is about vitality and vigor and energy. It is about excelling at the many challenges that face humans daily.

But how do we do it? How do we excel in life? By trying practices like the ones described in this jewel of a book. Here Kathy elegantly describes how health is a multidimensional experience of body, mind, and spirit and should be thought of as an ever-evolving process. As you try to make the small shifts and incremental changes she suggests, you will start to feel more conscious, more plugged in, more alive, and find yourself getting better and better at life.

The beauty of Kathy's approach is her understanding that everything we do has an internal effect. So being inauthentic or dishonest with others (and yourself) hurts you subconsciously—and physically. And wellness means not just that you don't have any particular illness or complaint but that you have abundant energy, exude a keen sense of purpose and place in the world, and consider the whole rather than just yourself.

How you eat, communicate, work out conflicts, and navigate your life should benefit not only you, but every other living being (including the planet we inhabit). This is a radical concept that will catch many of us off guard, but this is the ultimate holistic concept. Subtle influences on how we treat our world will have a multiplier effect on us, not just directly from reduction of pollution and global warming, but also because we become aware of our precious legacy—our bodies.

Kathy's work teaches us how to be healthy and happy, but *also* how to bring light and vitality to the "big picture" issues of interconnectedness, peace, and even love (an uncomfortable word for many healers). Awareness of the power that we have over our lives can catalyze a swift movement along the continuum of our evolution as individuals and as a people.

In fact, dealing with a health crisis or challenge can become an opportunity for us to hone our skills as healers, because ultimately we are all healers. By educating ourselves with some of the strategies Kathy offers, including adopting an attitude of "leaning into" wellness rather than forcing ourselves into strict regimens; building a momentum by adding gradually to our "bag of tricks" rather than imposing change too quickly; and using our personal power of choice—choosing to see and experience life at the highest levels of engagement and connection—we can, to a great extent, *create* wellness. Kathy reminds us that the important thing is simply to turn toward wellness and build, bit by bit, a certain momentum. Eventually a tipping point is reached and a real breakthrough—of body, mind, *and* spirit—can be ours.

Moreover, Kathy shows us that it's really a dance. As we grow in our own health and happiness, we contribute to an environment ripe for change. And finally, she reminds us that sometimes all we need to do is sit back and allow a mystical intercession to take place. By breaking things down into such manageable steps—steps that organically lead to breakthroughs of consciousness, connection, and health—Kathy has handed us the keys to "quantum wellness." What a gift.

It's up to us to decide to take the first step.

Mehmet Oz, M.D.
New York, New York

Quantum
Wellness

PART ONE

The Quantum Approach

CHAPTER ONE

What Is Quantum Wellness?
Making the Body-Mind-Spirit Connection

IF AN OLD FRIEND WERE TO GREET YOU ON THE STREET AND ASK, "How are you?" what would it take for you to answer honestly, "I'm very well, thank you"?

The truth is, many of us have no idea. We tend to think of being well as having no illness or trouble gnawing at us at that particular moment. We confuse wellness with an absence of something—a lack of pain or bodily complaints. But is that really wellness?

Or is wellness something far greater, far more exhilarating and alive? With this book, I hope to convince you that wellness is a condition involving every aspect of your being—body, mind, and spirit. That to be truly well means to be operating at full throttle no matter your age or position in life; to be in a constant dance of pushing past previous limits and breaking new ground. You feel like you are in the center of the vortex of life, filled with energy and a creative spark. You have a certain zip in your gait and a warm feeling of peace in your heart, and it is as if there is some supercharged energy flowing through you. You feel brilliantly alive and connected to everything that is.

Is this too much to ask, especially given the state of the nation, the global community, the planet?

3

Absolutely not.

And it isn't all that hard to do.

As I will show you in this book, wellness begins with paying attention to the little stuff, and then it swells in momentum until we find ourselves on a whole new playing field. We start by taking a look at our lives with honest eyes and then setting a few clear intentions to change. We take a small step here, and another there, and before we know it, we are made new.

You see, wellness is not so much a goal as a process, a journey, a way of orienting yourself toward life. It's a feeling of total participation that involves being in balance in the three key dimensions of body, mind, and spirit, and always looking at your actions and responses to life as they affect these three dimensions and are affected by them. It's about how you eat, how you listen to and take care of your body, how you process your feelings and connect to the larger world.

Yes, it is possible to achieve this state of wellness. I have done it, and I have helped or witnessed many other people doing it, too.

In this book, we will start small but we will always be holistic in our approach. For example, when I talk about eating, I'm going to look at food as a fuel that can support (or undermine) your body, your mind, *and* your spirit. I will also suggest a way of eating that does no harm to the rest of the planet. That may seem next to impossible. It's hard enough to get a healthy meal on the table without having to think about the environmental impact of every single thing on your plate. And when you have no time to begin with, you sometimes want to throw up your hands and grab a burger. But I will show you how possible it really is. You'll take some comfortable, small steps, develop a few new shopping and cooking habits—easy ones, delicious ones— and pretty soon you'll find yourself making healthier and healthier food choices all the time, without much effort at all.

The same goes for making room for feeling your feelings or tending to your spirit or your weight or your aches and pains. Small steps—simple changes to what you eat; a few new exercises; slight shifts in the way you perceive and resolve conflict, in the way you communicate; some gentle new practices to strengthen your spiritual life—followed by a few more small steps, and pretty soon you'll discover you've taken a quantum leap in how you feel and how you experience life.

The term *quantum* brings to mind several meanings. Primarily, it refers to very tiny particles and waves that are invisible to the naked eye. It also brings to mind a sudden leap from one virtual state into a new manifest state, as if a particular result had been plucked out of a sea of potentialities. And lastly, this leap, or spontaneous shift, is very much affected by the observer. So *quantum wellness,* to me, is about the tiny little things that we invest our energy in every day and every moment. These little investments of attention hold us in a steady and predictable place. But when we make shifts—no matter how small and subtle—we agitate the norm. And the more we turn our attention to wellness—to eating consciously (both for ourselves and for its comprehensive impact; more on that later), to resolving our interpersonal conflicts, to reducing our footprint, just to name a few—the more we stoke the fires of change. The momentum we generate through our actions leads, eventually, to a tipping point, and then there is a breakthrough, a quantum leap. We get to breakthrough levels of wellness by turning our attention to those things that add to the force field of wellness.

Quantum wellness is not about imposing big changes but about leaning into wellness, comfortably, adding things here and there to the thrust and taking baby steps toward the changes we want to achieve.

Think about it. This happens in life all the time. Maybe you are someone who used to be anxious all the time, relying on antianx-iety medication to get through the day, and then one day realized that you hadn't taken your medication for a while and you were just fine. (By the way, I don't recommend going off any medication with-out the help or advice of a health-care professional.) You aren't sure if it was the exercise regimen that soothed your nerves or the new friends you chose to be around or the fact that you gave up drinking caffeine. All you know is that you are not a wreck any-more. Or maybe you were like me and had acne for as long as you could remember, but then woke up one morning with clear skin and never had so much as another blemish. I'm not sure if I just grew through the hormonal period or if my skin looks better because I changed my diet and drink more water. In each of these examples, there were lots of little changes made, but something big and mon-umental resulted.

These shifts reshape our lives. Of course, they don't come out of nowhere: they're not magic. We have to do the footwork to make them happen. But it's the small, incremental changes that vault us to a new experience of ourselves. Remember that as you approach this work.

So *how* do quantum leaps happen? And can we help them hap-pen? Can we be more in control of them so that we can create trans-formation in our lives? Good questions.

The fact is, we don't really know the very specifics of how a quan-tum leap happens per se, and that tends to make us nervous. Even the greatest of quantum physicists doesn't really understand the ex-act mechanism. But the point is, they do happen. The implication here is that we too can affect the probability of something spectac-ular materializing by the energy we put into supporting the new.

No, this doesn't mean we can hold in our mind a picture of a 24-inch waist and then suddenly shrink. That would be magical thinking. Quantum thinking isn't about kicking back and doing nothing, it's about understanding the incredible power of consciousness and choice. And doing things with relative ease.

Don't worry. No one is suggesting that you relinquish your worldly love of "stuff" or move to a mountaintop in order to be a more spiritual person; you can be conscious while also enjoying the things that make you happy. Quantum wellness isn't about deprivation and it's not about perfection. It is about pointing yourself in the direction of growth, training yourself to get comfortable with your highest potential, and then taking small steps to support that shift. It's about showing up for yourself, day by day, and then one day finding that you've undergone a transformation.

I have been at this self-improvement game for a long time and have spent many (too many) years trying to follow guidelines and stick to rules put forth by various gurus. But I always ended up feeling like a failure. When I ate too much sugar, I crucified myself, which of course made me eat even more. When I missed too many days of exercise, I fell into slothful periods that sometimes lasted for months. If I wasn't meditating regularly, I figured I was just not cut out for the spiritual life and gave up. By being so demanding of myself, I ended up getting nowhere; the do-or-die approach definitely did not work with me.

And then I discovered that change and growth are part of our nature. We just have to point ourselves in the right direction and start moving toward what it is we want to manifest. We have to accept where we are and make peace with it, and we'll find the strength and the will to change. I know that's how it worked for me.

When I made the decision to accept myself as I was, I began to eat better, exercise regularly, and do all the things I had always wanted to do. It wasn't that it just happened by itself, but it happened naturally and without too much stress. And now, looking back, I can see that I was taking four simple steps:

1. **Listen and learn.**
2. **Set an intention.**
3. **Come up with a plan.**
4. **Make the move.**

For example, I used to smoke a pack of cigarettes a day. I tried so many times to quit: I drenched the pack with water so I couldn't retrieve the cigarettes. I did acupuncture to foil the desire. I wore a patch. I underwent hypnosis. Nothing worked. So I just gave up and said, "Okay, this is where I am now." All the while I kept reading about what nicotine does to the body and how smoking hurts your lungs and immune system. Not to mention how it ages your skin.

I just listened and learned. I didn't resist the information; I simply took it in (while still smoking) and let it settle into my mind.

Then I set my intention to be a nonsmoker. I didn't know how I would get there, because I had failed so many times, but I just put it out there to the world that I wanted to be a person who smelled good and enjoyed downtime without jonesing for the next drag. I didn't beat myself up every time I lit up, but I *did* think about the information I had downloaded. And I began to feel my energy moving in the direction of healing, just trusting that I would get there. After a few months of this, I came up with a plan to attend a smoking-cessation workshop, which I would follow with a week's vacation away by myself. Once again I put it out into the ether that I was ready and willing to act when the time felt right.

Three days later I was flipping through a neighborhood periodical and came across an ad that seemed to jump off the page for a "stop smoking" class, and I made my move.

This whole process—from gathering information to going away on a solo vacation—probably lasted six months, but it stuck because I simply allowed myself to be where I was and to go at my own pace. Had I tried to do it all in one grandiose move, I probably would have fallen back into my old habit, but since I saw myself on a path, I felt comfortable just nudging myself gradually in the right direction.

We are all at various points along the continuum of wellness; we arrive at and handle different junctures according to our own personal comfort levels. We may be ahead of the game in physical fitness while lagging behind in spiritual awareness, or very emotionally and psychologically astute but lazy in the way we eat. It's all okay. We just have to be willing to be honest with ourselves about where we are and then work to bring ourselves up to speed wherever growth is needed.

We can hasten our progress by taking an honest inventory and then mapping out where we'd like to go. For me and my nicotine addiction, I knew there was a better way to live, and I wanted to move in the direction of being free of the habit. At the same time I very much wanted to keep doing what I was doing. I loved the social bonding with other smokers; I loved the ritual of settling into the day with a smoke to get my adrenaline flowing. But I also knew I couldn't advance in my life—physically or emotionally—without dealing with my attachment to a bad dependency. I knew where I was on my continuum and decided it was time to press onward.

After I quit, my life took a leap forward. I began to work with cancer patients, teaching them guided meditation and breathing exercises, not as a direct result of quitting smoking, but more as part of a "grand plan" for my life. I certainly couldn't have taken that direction had I remained a smoker. No one wants to smell smoke on their counselor; and who would have believed I knew what I was talking about if I couldn't even shed my own unhealthy habit? The point is, once I followed through on my decision to change in one area of my life, other areas also experienced a major shift. I went from being a barely working model to being a writer and counselor. Quitting smoking had always seemed nearly impossible, but I accomplished it by staying relaxed about it, taking very doable steps, and allowing myself to be directed by an inner compass. I showed up as a willing participant in my own conscious evolution, let the momentum build, and the rest unfolded with and for me.

Our development is an unfinished and ongoing story. That's what is so exciting; we are creating ourselves and our world as we go. And every little move we make, each decision and perception we land on, makes a difference in how things unfold.

Imagine yourself standing at the edge of a pond. The water is calm, placid, and smooth like glass. In your hand, you hold a pebble. You drop the pebble into the water, and from the place where the pebble submerges, ripples ruffle the water's surface. The small waves start at the point of the pebble's entry, and they make their way the entire distance to the banks of the pond, touching the earth in waves.

You are the pond, and every thought, action, and feeling is a pebble, influencing your body, relationships, future, and present moment. In your existence, there is no insignificant moment. The universe is also that pond, and you are that pebble. Your life, energy, and love echo energetically to the very edges of all creation. You have that much power.

To help you understand this critical point, we can look to an interesting discovery made in meteorology called the butterfly effect. In 1961, Edward Norton Lorenz entered a figure for wind velocity into a computer in an attempt to predict weather conditions. Taking a shortcut, he entered .506 instead of .506127. What he found was astounding: that tiny difference of .000127 radically altered the ensuing weather scenario. The concept Lorenz developed around his findings became known as the butterfly effect, because a wind velocity difference of .000127 seems so totally insignificant—much like the difference in velocity that might be caused by the flapping wings of a butterfly. Lorenz concluded that the slightest and seemingly most insignificant initial condition could drastically modify the weather going forward. That tiny variation could create such a different path or momentum, that it might in fact initiate a chain of meteorological events that could change a sunny day into a tornado. In chaos theory, this is known as sensitive dependence on initial conditions. A tiny shift matters that much. The message is obvious, and I find the metaphorical conclusion—that every action, no matter how small, can cause a huge reaction somewhere else or at some future time—to be profound (and true).

The more we adjust or shift—even in tiny ways—the more we can look forward to sweeping changes showing up in our lives. We can cut one thing out of our diet, add a minute or two of meditation, or turn our attention just for a moment toward kindness, and before we know it we are different people creating a different world. This far-reaching shift is dependent entirely on our willingness to consistently move along the wellness continuum, in whatever incremental ways we can.

In the atmosphere, as in life, every small factor is significant and influential. This is why setting your intention and living your life in a way that pulls you toward your ultimate empowerment—in every moment—is so important. You can direct your experience of life in such a fundamental way. Every conversation you have, every morsel you eat, every purchase you make, and on and on, factors in to where you will find yourself in a week, a year, or a decade.

A friend of mine likes to remind me that even just wearing a button or putting a bumper sticker on your car *can* change the course of history. That's not just hyperbole. Think about it. Say the button sparks a conversation in the checkout line in the supermarket. The person you chatted with then adopts the change you are promoting. You have just changed every remaining day of that person's life. And if that person decides to make that advocacy issue his life's mission, well then, his excitement will generate yet more new waves in the world (or pond!) and thus the dance of life takes a new twist! All from simply putting a bumper sticker on your car or wearing a button.

Every little thing you do adds up and before you know it you've created your life. And how you create your life ripples out and affects everyone and everything that crosses your path, known or unknown to you.

Now imagine that you are in a rowboat, and everything you do is one push of the paddle. Is it a strong stroke, moving you forward? Or is it sideways or chaotic, leaving you vulnerable to the current? Think of this wellness journey as that rowboat. Once you get the hang of rowing with the current and not against it, in harmony with who you truly are at your highest potential, every move you make will move you forward with greater efficiency. Just follow the rhythm of the current, add to it some of your own muscle, and you'll soon be amazed at how your momentum increases and you start meeting and surpassing your goals.

As you awaken to this power to affect your life, pay close attention to your feelings and observations. Ask yourself: Where am I now and where do I want to be? Just be aware. The more you become aware of the effects of each choice you make, the more you will be able to choose differently and better for yourself. As you live more creatively, you'll be amazed at how these small moments come together and inform your big breakthroughs.

Body, mind, and spirit all work together to create wellness, and we simply cannot experience the upsurge, the full thrust required for a quantum shift when any of these three areas goes unheeded. We can go to the gym every day and eat the right foods, but if our souls are sick, we won't be well. We can meditate till the cows come home and yet not feel quite right in our bodies if we are still smoking or eating sugar or feeling belittled at work. But don't worry: being imperfect is all part of the process. We don't have to be masterful. We need not get everything just right. We just need to push ourselves a little bit here and there to get the momentum going, and from that, strength and confidence will settle into the parts of us that lag behind. And then the magic happens: momentous changes occur seemingly on their own. Look at it this way: all the bits and pieces of our lives fit and flow together like an ever-shifting matrix of influences. We are in constant formation, and there comes a moment—unchosen and unforeseeable by us—when everything just clicks, and a leap occurs.

An organism or species evolves through multiple and simultaneous changes. Our musculature—both intellectual and biological—must be worked on even as our spiritual sights are raised. And everything goes into the creative—or evolutionary—soup. We throw in a bit of this, stir in a bit of that—until we find we've created something new for ourselves.

The game is about learning how to evolve more and more efficiently, building on each tiny transcendent moment until we reach a tipping point. And then the breakthrough happens. Once you begin to pay attention to the interplay of your physical, emotional, and spiritual health and then set an intention to change, change will come. Incrementally and, ultimately, with breathtaking clarity. I guarantee it.

How to Use This Book

I like to use a cross-training metaphor when it comes to working on wellness. Just as we would work simultaneously on our strength, endurance, flexibility, and gross motor skills in order to become better athletes, throughout this book we will take a cross-training approach to health and wellness, using tools such as self-examination, exercise, cleaning up your diet, spiritual inner work, journaling, and, yes, having fun (!) to address whatever might be bothering you physically, emotionally, or spiritually. This only makes sense, doesn't it? If the issues that affect how we feel are multidimensional, their resolution must be, too.

Whether you are feeling sluggish or disconnected or are coping with a serious chronic illness, you will find a mix of practices and ideas here, in the interplay of which you will experience your wellness breakthroughs. The tools are effective on their own, but two or more used together will make the whole process more effective, more rapid, and more fun. Also, if you mix things up you won't get bored or overwhelmed.

You will also discover how each tool supports the other realms. The better you feel physically, for example, the more fun you will want to have; having more fun, you will naturally be inclined to look for ways to share your joy. You will also experience a broader view of yourself and the world around you.

I once heard Ken Wilber, the highly acclaimed transpersonal philosopher, describe a study in which one group of people learned to meditate under the tutelage of a monk. Their focus was singular and intense as the monk coached them and guided them to learn a certain method. The other group of meditation students, also overseen by the monk, simultaneously undertook a weight-lifting program. These students divided their time between learning to improve *both* skills. Guess who progressed more in their meditation practice? Not the students who stayed singularly focused; they learned and progressed, but not nearly as much as the students who spread their energy between the two endeavors. Wilber explains that by engaging your multiple intelligences (whether musical, mathematical, intuitive, or as yet undefined) you light up different areas of the brain, creating more space for a broader breakthrough.

By approaching your wellness goals in a multipronged way, you will become more proficient all around. Remember, we are made up of multiple moving parts; we vary in levels of spiritual aptitude as well as emotional and intellectual astuteness. We also have physical abilities that range from poor to excellent. Just observe where you think you could improve, and choose the tool or practice that will help you get there.

I encourage you to read through each chapter and try a few ideas that you think would make the most difference. Don't try tackling all of them at once; rather, gain some mastery of one or two until you feel comfortable, and then add another into the mix. By building your toolbox slowly and organically, you construct a launchpad from upon which this whole cross-training approach can take wing.

As you embark on a journey toward quantum wellness, you can count on two things:

1. As you increase your knowledge of what it is to be well, everything that is "not well" will reveal itself. You will be more readily able to identify that which needs your attention.

2. You will find within you the ability to bring light to all those places that are wounded or unenlightened so that you can experience magnificent multidimensional wellness.

You see, the path of wellness is a path of transcendence. You will constantly be brought to the walls that keep you stuck and you will be challenged to overcome them. You will become more attuned to all the wonder and grace at work in the world today—the miraculous cures, the everyday heroes who have stepped out of their comfort zone and made a difference, the stories of human kindness that would melt any heart. As you undertake to become more and more well, you will find yourself resonating more with that extraordinary energy. In fact, you will, through your own magnetic, amped-up vitality, draw to you events, meetings, and circumstances that you might never have imagined possible.

It is said that as you rise, the world rises to greet you. As you strive toward greater levels of wellness, you will discover that you are not working alone or in a void; you are part of a larger whole that is also leaning forward into life. You will intuit what is right while at the same time being guided toward the next steps. You will be carried along even as you push yourself toward greater and greater levels of happiness and health.

Each of us has a part in this process. We are all meant to become free, whole, and healed. A few steps along the wellness continuum and you will no longer be at a loss for words when someone asks you, "How are you today?"

Please join me as we explore the simple changes and small steps that will lead you to quantum wellness.

CHAPTER TWO

The Eight Pillars of Wellness

OVER THE YEARS I HAVE FOUND EIGHT AREAS OF PRACTICE THAT ARE particularly powerful and compatible for wellness cross-training. They are:

- meditation
- visualization
- fun activities
- conscious eating
- exercise
- self-work
- spiritual practice
- service

Before you panic, I am not suggesting that you use all eight all the time, only that you think of wellness as something truly multi-faceted, and that you remain open to the idea that most of the issues we face in life, be they physical, emotional, or what have you, have their roots *and* their resolution not just in one dimension but in several.

My friend Janet comes to mind here. She is a successful businesswoman who had a lifelong struggle with her weight. As much as she understands calories and the need for exercise, over the years her weight fluctuated wildly. Sometimes she was thin, feeling confident and victorious. And then she would hit some snag in her life and put on 50 pounds. She tried every diet in the book, and they each seemed to work for a while. She went to therapy and talked about her feelings and why she might be hiding behind the weight. And she even worked at visualizing herself as fit and happy. But these subtler methods never had immediate or lasting enough results, and she would end up throwing up her hands and reverting to the old, self-sabotaging behavior of indulging her cravings.

It was only when Janet decided that she didn't want to eat anything that caused harm to another creature that things made a permanent turn for the better. Her diet was no longer a "diet" but a conscious choice to be kinder. This little decision boosted her confidence in herself and replaced her old deprivation thinking with a sense of joyful discipline. And when Janet added back in some of the practices she had tried before—visualizing, exercising, and introspection—the "soup" of it all pushed her over the edge.

She is now thin and fit and has been for over ten years. Not because of one magic-bullet solution, but because she kept at her process until one tiny decision made it all come together and work in a whole new way. That's how quantum wellness works.

I encourage you to read through my description of each of the eight practices and decide on a few that you think would make the most difference for you right now. Master a few and then add in a new one when you feel ready. By building your wellness toolbox slowly and organically, you will build the kind of strong foundation upon which the whole cross-training approach can flourish and bring you truly amazing results.

A Wellness Checkup

First, let's check in and see what's going on for you right now. What is happening in your life that is keeping you from feeling like you are at your peak? Are you in conflict in any of your relationships? Do you get enough sleep? Do you have good ways of handling whatever stresses you out in life? Are you living with aches and pains that have just become your idea of normal? Or maybe you don't have any concerns or complaints right now. If that's the case, look at the little things you'd like to be able to change or resolve. We all have our burdens— be they physical, financial, interpersonal, or emotional—and checking in with ourselves and really listening to what comes up are the first steps toward our quantum leap to wellness.

Right now, ask yourself:

- *What is bothering me most right now?* Think of physical symptoms but also consider your general emotional state.

- *What do I think are the material (real world or physical) causes?* What have you tried? What works and what doesn't?

- *What are the emotional components?* How can you address this area?

- *Is there a spiritual lesson my higher Self is trying to teach me?* Have you taken in the lesson or are you resisting it?

Just let yourself roll the questions around for a bit. Here is an example of how the thought process might go:

- **What is bothering me most right now?**

I am having heart palpitations and I don't know if it is serious or not. I get very sweaty and cold and my heart seems to be beating erratically. It usually happens in the middle of the night. At times my chest feels so tight I think I must surely be having a heart attack, but I'm not, because the cardiologist checked me twice, and there is no sign of a heart attack. This has been going on for a few weeks. I'm really scared that something terrible is going to happen.

- **What do I think is the material cause? What have I tried? What works and what doesn't?**

I've heard that being low on potassium and magnesium could cause heart palpitations. So I've taken supplements and it seems to help but not cure the situation. Maybe I was drinking too much coffee, but I don't think that's the sole reason. I've since given up caffeine, and that too might be helping. Still, that hasn't stopped it from happening altogether.

- **What are the emotional components? How can I address this area?**

I really don't like being told that this could be an anxiety attack or stress induced. I resent not being taken seriously by my doctors. Still, I have to wonder if perhaps the pressure I've been under isn't affecting me after all. My money concerns have been weighing seriously on me; work seems to be drying up and I have so many unpaid bills. My credit cards are over the moon. I'm angry that no one is stepping in to help me and I have my kids to feed and send to school. I'm really scared that if I don't figure out the next step, we'll end up losing the house. Hmm, I guess I do have a lot of stress and anxiety. Maybe I can do some breathing exercises to relax. And I think I will check out the Debtors Anonymous group that I saw was free and open to the public. Perhaps I can scale down my life to ease the financial burden I'm feeling. Already, just thinking this through, I feel better. Clearly, I have to deal with some emotional stuff if I want to be symptom-free.

- **Is there a spiritual lesson my higher Self is trying to teach me? Am I resisting it?**

Now that I think about it, I realize that I had to get pretty alarmed before I woke up and snapped out of this negative habituation of stress, anger, and overspending. I think this happened so that I would look at what needs to change in my life. There are fundamental things that I need to address: I have to look at my anger and see how I'm perpetuating it. I have to realize that nothing is going to change until I change. And I have to think about what is important—my family, my health, my serenity—and do the work that will support those things. I'm really glad this health crisis happened. I see now that there was a purpose and I'm glad I paid attention. I can already feel my chest relaxing and my heart resuming a normal rhythm.

As you spend some time really listening to yourself, focusing on each aspect of body, mind, and spirit, you will come to see the whole picture of your state of being and begin to intuit what you need to

21

do. You will see that you have a natural inclination to heal and you will feel more comfortable in lending your conscious awareness to the process.

We are human; we have all sorts of shortcomings and challenges. Some of us have robust health and fragile emotions; some of us have just the opposite. The better we come to know and accept ourselves, the more well and wise we will become. At this point, you don't have to do anything except simply be aware of what's going on inside you. Get to know your body, understand your mind, and embrace your spiritual path. Once you connect the dots, the next steps will become apparent.

The Cross-Training Practices

Meditation is a word that scares a lot of people. They don't think they're the "kind of person" who could possibly sit for long stretches with an empty mind. I'm not asking you to do that. Meditation, as I use the word, is simply a state of quiet contemplation. It involves turning your focus inward for at least a few moments at a time so you can access a deeper reality.

Practicing a daily ritual of meditation almost always leads to positive changes in your life in that you are more relaxed and "in tune" throughout the day and can better handle stress and adversity. You are more present to life and can respond in a more balanced and thoughtful way to the situations that come up.

Some people meditate as a means to commune with Spirit, while others use meditation as a technique to cultivate mental discipline. Whatever the goal, the physiological effects of meditation are many: change in metabolism due to the lowering of biochemical by-products of stress, lowered heart rate and blood pressure, and greater ease of respiration. When you meditate, there is an increase in activity in the left prefrontal cortex of your brain, the area associated with the ability to focus and concentrate, plan, and enjoy positive feelings. Studies indicate that meditators also tend to have less depression and anxiety.

Try this:

To meditate, all you have to do is find a private and comfortable place to close your eyes. Sit on a cushion cross-legged (resting attentively in a chair or lying on your back is fine too, if that will persuade you to do it!) and take in ten nice breaths. Listen to the sound of the air as it enters and exits your nose. Breathing through your nose stimulates what in yoga are called *nadi*—subtle channels of life force. By activating these channels, you not only calm the nervous system but also stir up the *prana,* or vitality, flowing through your body.

As you inhale, imagine a beautiful grace-filled light entering into the top of your head, and upon exhaling, picture sharing that light with the world. See the breath making a loop as it comes in and goes out. Keep your practice simple by repeating a mantra (a word or phrase that inspires you). A few that I use are: "Peace," "Yes," or "I am here." Saying a mantra will help pull you back to the energy you want to focus on.

Try not to breathe so deeply that you hyperventilate, but rather bring the air all the way down to your belly and back up through your chest. Start off by taking ten breaths and gradually work your way up to a twenty-minute meditation as you get more used to cycling down and relaxing. Ease into it just as you would ease into an exercise program. You can use a kitchen timer or gently open your eyes from time to time to check on how many minutes you have left.

This is just one way to meditate—a kind of all-purpose method. There are many other forms of meditation, and it's a good idea to explore until you find a method that works for you. Teachers and classes can guide you into a practice; these days you can find meditation in yoga studios, churches, temples, and monasteries. Find what feels right and then just keep showing up. Even if you think you are too restless, close your eyes for just a few minutes (or the ten breaths) and go inside. As often as you can, keep coming back to the present moment and invest your energy in experiencing the depth that meditation offers.

Visualization is more active than meditation. It is a way of mapping out the changes and upgrades you wish to make. You see, the neurocircuitry in our brains holds all the messages we have received repeatedly throughout our lives, and most especially the ones we received in the formative years of childhood. It's as if each meaningful event or exchange with someone cut a groove into our thinking, and with each experience that supported that message the groove became deeper and more firmly entrenched. Repetition, strong emotion or sensation, trauma, or resistance—these all affect our hard wiring, influencing our emotional circuitry. We respond to new situations on the basis of this circuitry, and it often prevents us from experiencing all the joy and vitality that is our birthright.

For instance, if your parents always told you (repetition) you were not very smart, you would probably come to agree with them and see yourself as not so smart. Or if you had your first orgasm (strong emotion or sensation) with someone who was domineering and direct, domineering and direct personalities would probably always feel sexy to you. Or if you were molested as a child (trauma), you might firmly believe that you were never safe no matter where you were or who you were with.

On the other hand, if you were taught that anger was bad, you might live your life desperately trying to resist (resistance) or deny your anger. But the irony is that when we resist something we actually energize it. In this case, your disowned anger remains embedded in your field of energy. Resistance takes a lot of energy.

We all project our deeply held and sometimes unconscious beliefs out into the world, and the world mirrors back to us more of the same. Basically, we get stuck in a rut because our response to new situations depends on emotions experienced or patterns set up in the past.

In order to shake things up, you have to shake loose your mindset. If you want to change the way you are feeling, you have to repattern your energy and literally create a new neurocircuitry. That's where visualization comes in. In visualizing, you feed your brain new images to replace the embedded ones, and these then lay new circuits. This is sometimes called guided imagery. And it works. (If you are interested in the science behind guided imagery, see the Suggested Reading and Viewing section at the back of this book.)

Think of your mind as a toy train set. The train (your thoughts) goes round and round the same track (negative images) until you build on to your train set a new track (fresh image and new potential) and pull the switch for it to transfer over (upgraded thought system). The old tracks are still there, but you have just given yourself some new routes to travel. That's what visualization does. It changes your course. It upgrades your mind-set by providing a new map for where you want your energy to go. And as you learn to switch up the images of yourself, everything else follows. You start gravitating more toward experiences and practices that support the new images.

This is a big part of how a quantum leap happens. We witness or observe (visualize) ourselves with a different eye, and thus jump-start the process of upgrading our state of wellness.

Visualization helps you rejigger the way you see things so that you can respond to life differently; it takes apart old images and replaces them with new and better ones. With these new images in place, you will begin to think differently, and as you think and behave differently, people will change the way they respond to you.

If you stand up straight, for instance, because you have visualized yourself as healthy and confident, people will most likely see you as capable and attractive—and will treat you accordingly. Which will reinforce that self-image. See how the cycle of cause and effect kicks in? How you see yourself is how people will see you; what you project out into the world starts with how you experience yourself inside. First in your mind, then in the material world. This shift informs how you relate to people and affects your choices on many levels (if you visualize yourself as happy, you might naturally smile more; when you smile, your mood naturally lifts) and so on. Before you know it, you will experience life—your health and well-being—at a whole new level. Sometimes the differences are subtle, and sometimes they are massive.

Visualization helps us clarify what we want and gives us the map to get there. If, for instance, you want to eat healthier but see yourself as someone who could never have the discipline to stick to a good plan, you can replace that picture with one of someone who loves and craves healthy food. Imagine feeling robust and energetic. See yourself eating well and enjoying it. Where you invest your attention is where the energy flows; it's all about creating a new structure.

The crazy thing is, the brain literally does not know the difference between what is real and what is imagined. You've probably heard of the experiment in which a person pictures biting into a lemon, and even though there is no such lemon, the person puckers his lips. The brain triggered a real and physical response simply from a conjured image. Material reality started from a thought—an idea that was nuanced and enhanced by conscious imagination—and then a real physical response manifested. Try it!

So if you give yourself enough new information, you will begin to shift your consciousness. And then your actions will reflect and follow that shift. If we hold the image—and we *always* hold images whether we are aware of it or not—of ourselves as sluggish or gluttonous, with no willpower, our stomach rumbles for something "bad" and we can't stop thinking about it until we've polished off enough to feel guilty and ashamed, and round and round we go. Once we perceive ourselves differently, all else follows.

The quantum leap—the actual physical change—is largely influenced by a shift in perception. Of yourself, and of the way things work.

Try this:

"I Am Healthy, Happy, and Transformed"
A Basic Visualization Technique
Here is a visualization technique I have used for many years with people who claim to be unable to reach their goals. It helps them change the images in their mind, and things begin shifting in the external world soon thereafter. For instance, if you have always (consciously or unconsciously) held to the image that relationships are difficult and disappointing, it is likely that you will draw to yourself difficult and disappointing relationships. But if you practice visualizing a relationship that is easy and joyful, you are far more likely to attract a partner who can make that kind of relationship with you.

Read through the practice first to get the general idea, and then close your eyes and use your imagination to make it as real as possible. If you want, you can record yourself reading the words and then play them back, letting your mind totally relax into the new imagery.

Breathing slowly and deeply, retreat into the deeper regions of your mind.

Notice all the thoughts and images bustling about and just allow them to be there.

See yourself as you are now. Try not to judge, but simply be with that person who is doing the best she can.

Now let that image fade into the background. If it doesn't want to go away, it's okay; just let it hang around.

Begin to conjure up in your mind's eye an image of yourself thriving and enjoying your life. Notice the sound of laughter, the colors of happiness. Watch as you flow through your days making excellent decisions that support wellness in all areas of your body, mind, and spirit.

See yourself eating conscientiously and loving the fact that you have turned a corner. See yourself being active, taking quiet time, and enjoying a heightened level of creativity. See that everything you do benefits not only you but also every living thing on the planet.

Notice how people gravitate toward you and events seem to work out effortlessly and in your favor. There is synchronicity and magic in the air.

Sense that there is now a brilliant energy infused into everything you do. Your life has new purpose to it. You feel elevated and very connected to the essence of life itself.

Feel in each and every cell of your body that you are lifted and made new. Relax into the comfort of knowing that all is well.

Breathe deeply ten more times as you emanate the deep gratitude that flows from your heart. You are firmly and joyfully on your path.

When you are ready, open your eyes.

This kind of rewiring of your mind has the potential to bring about sudden changes. Again, this isn't hocus-pocus. You can't simply think something and then have it be so. The repatterning of your mind must be followed up by solid action steps. You have to change your behavior. But the changes don't have to be grand or dramatic. They just have to be moving in the direction of your own growth and wellness.

For instance, when I imagined myself being happy and well, I had the sense that I was being cleaned and purified, almost as if I were being rinsed. The steps I took in "real life" that supported this image were (1) I began drinking a lot more water and (2) I decided to go on a cleanse (more on that later) at least once a year and (3) I also cleaned out my closets and took a hard look at some dusty relationships that needed to be addressed. The imagery exercise primed me for cleansing on various levels, but then I took some steps to really manifest it.

Doing guided imagery work is certainly not a one-time deal; it's something you can do as often as you think about it. You really want to continue fortifying (without clinging to) the new images that are taking root in your consciousness. I recommend that people close their eyes and let their minds create at least once a day. As with any new exercise or program, start gradually (spend even just a minute), and practice often. For me, I prefer to flash on the images many times throughout the day rather than sit and focus for a long period of time. But do what feels right to you.

A note here: it is absolutely critical that you don't constantly look to see when and how things are manifesting. This kind of constant evaluation (is it working yet? why am I not seeing results yet?) sets back what is supposed to be a process of initiation and release. Your job is to initiate the shift by putting your mind in a new place and then letting go, releasing the details of how it actually unfolds to the ether. When you are always looking for the results (why don't I have clearer skin yet? why hasn't the irritation gone away yet?), you are sending out pushy and needy energy. My message is this: do your work, and then let go. Relax and assume the right things will come to pass.

Transformation happens in its own time; you can take the steps to prepare for it, but then it's best to step aside and allow for that mysterious grace to take over. That's how quantum leaps in wellness work.

Fun activities. This one often surprises people, but I can't imagine being well without having any fun. Fun activities, whatever they might be for you, bring levity to your life. They loosen up your energy and bring in optimism. They remind you that life is meant to be joyful. You can go to a club (without the agenda to meet someone) and dance for a few hours, regularly show up for a game of basketball or tennis or whatever you fancy, paint something wild and colorful, or lose yourself in your hobby of choice. Play with your kids or run on the beach with your dogs and watch them have the time of their life.

One of the ways I have fun is I get in my car and drive a beautiful stretch of road between Los Angeles and Big Sur and blast my favorite songs. If anyone saw me singing along at the top of my lungs, I'm sure they would think I'd lost my mind. But these are some of my most ecstatic moments, moments when I feel positively carried by magic.

In whatever you do for fun, see the simple blessing in being able to be so happy. Feel the gratitude that comes with appreciating the fullness of life. When you laugh at a funny movie or get silly with friends, you can feel the weight of all your responsibilities just slipping away. By taking your fun seriously, you will regain the quality of innocence in your life. Planning a fun activity gives you something to look forward to and then a precious memory to fondly look back on. Sometimes when you are trying to work on your health, you forget that the most important thing is to love life. If things get too serious or strenuous, you will feel overwhelmed and lose momentum. Just make a habit of doing something really fun and lighthearted at least once a day; those moments or hours of sheer delight will keep lifting your level of energy for the rest of the week.

Conscious eating. I'll be delving into the subject of food and eating in a couple of upcoming chapters, but for now let's just say it's crucial for your overall wellness that you give your body good fuel and that you bring awareness to your food choices. Eating consciously means not eating something just because it tastes good, and not blindly accepting that certain foods are good for you simply because they are marketed that way. Instead, it's about looking more closely at where your food comes from and how it got to your plate and choosing to eat foods that support life—all life, not just your own.

When you eat something, you take in the energy that went into creating that food. If the persons handling the food were possessed with resignation, disgust, anger, and fear that vibration is passed on to you when you ingest the product of their work. On the other hand, if you shop and consume consciously, making sure that to the best of your knowledge the workers who produced the items were fairly treated and the food was raised and harvested thoughtfully and for the good of all, you are more likely to take in the positive energy of peace, abundance, and harmony. Nutrition isn't just biochemical; it's also coded with the energy that goes into it. Once again, wellness is something to be mastered on all levels of body, mind, and spirit. Hence, the fresher, more peacefully handled, less-processed food will pass along a higher vibration. The food being sold today is all too often devoid of the consideration of how it affects us—and the world—holistically, and thus we remain a hungry, malnourished, prone-to-illness people.

Keep your eyes open and scrutinize the process from beginning to end; remain aware of how your dietary choices affect others. Eat in a way that is not only good for you but also good for everyone involved in bringing it to you: the farmers, the laborers and truck drivers, the animals, and the environment. And perhaps offer a moment of gratitude—whether silently and to yourself or out loud with your family—before a meal: *I rejoice in the abundance of this food. May my body be strengthened and my soul be nourished by the gift of it. And may every aspect of this food be blessed and filled with love.*

Exercise is a way of achieving fitness across the board in each of the arenas of body, mind, and spirit. By maintaining a moderate amount of exercise in your daily life (at least 30 minutes three to six times a week), you can significantly improve your overall well-being. The merits range from helping to prevent or alleviate the symptoms of major health conditions (such as cancer, heart disease, diabetes, and obesity) to improving your confidence and self-esteem. After a rigorous session of weight training or a fairly strenuous hike or walk, you can feel the circulation of energy throughout your entire system. Instead of feeling exhausted afterward, you actually feel energized and more alert.

First, for the physical benefits: When you exercise until you're breathing heavily, the respiratory system is improved by the deep rhythmic inhaling and exhaling. Your huffing and puffing helps the lungs increase their capacity to take in more oxygen, which then nourishes your cells and alkalizes your body.

When you breathe deeply, you relax your nervous system. Your blood also travels more efficiently to distribute essential nutrients throughout your entire system. And when you sweat, your perspiration detoxifies your body, helping to rinse out of your system all sorts of impurities that otherwise might have lingered.

Cardiovascular exercise is very beneficial in that it makes your heart a stronger and more capable muscle, better able to handle life's stresses and strains. The resting heart rate of someone who exercises is slower because less effort is needed to pump the blood; low blood pressure and a low resting heart rate are signs of good health.

Strength training is now said to be one of the best things you can do for your body. Whereas we used to think aerobic exercise was the thing to do, now studies show that if we push too hard for too long, the body starts to break down. Instead, we should do around 20 minutes to an hour of a brisk workout to get our heart pumping (to the point where you're breathing hard but can still carry on a conversation; if you can't talk, you are working too hard) and then focus more on resistance training.

It is said that muscles are the engine of youth; indeed, when you undertake a good program of lifting weights a few times a week, it turns back your physiological age by about 12 years. This kind of exercise is very effective in preventing osteoporosis (a weakening of the bones), because when you lift heavy weights you force your bones to adapt to the exertion placed on them by producing matrix proteins, which fortify them. Your muscles, tendons, and ligaments also become stronger, making your body better able to protect itself from the stresses that cause injury. Weight training also increases your metabolism, because as your muscles get bigger, your body uses up more calories even at rest.

Exercises such as yoga and tai chi require you to use your focus to maintain balance and concentration while increasing your coordination. Because proper breathing is such a key component, these sorts of exercises help to lower both heart rate and blood pressure. You can improve your posture and dexterity while working on your range of motion and flexibility; it is said in yogic tradition that a flexible spine is the key to youth and vitality because the life force (*prana*) can move freely and easily through a supple spine. Think of how a tree weathers a storm; it bends with the wind without breaking. Yoga has been known to balance and nourish the endocrine system as well as normalize the gastrointestinal function because certain nerve endings are stimulated when the body strikes particular poses. It is a science that has been practiced for thousands of years, and its aim is to unite the body, mind, and spirit. Yoga and its sister practices of the martial arts teach you to hone your bodily awareness and focus your attention in a singular and almost meditative way.

Most forms of exercise increase the muscle-to-fat ratio, making you leaner and stronger. Overall, exercise enhances your performance of everyday tasks and makes you feel good about yourself. Anxiety and depression are eased because working out stimulates the production of endorphins, which produce the feeling of well-being. Endorphins also combat the effects of cortisol, the stress hormone that wreaks havoc on the body. These neurotransmitters also provide natural pain relief and help you to feel at ease. Adrenaline, serotonin, and dopamine are other brain chemicals whose levels are raised by intense strength training or prolonged aerobic exercise; each contributes to feelings of energy, clarity, and alertness.

And not only does a good workout improve your sense of well-being, but it also improves your reaction time, mental acuity, and math skills. In fact, according to Dr. Dean Ornish, "Research is showing that exercise . . . may even help you grow so many new brain cells (a process called neurogenesis) that your brain actually gets bigger." The region that is most affected and grows the most is the hippocampus, which involves memory and cognition; in other words, exercise can make you smarter! So, if you want to feel happy, at ease, and clever, if you want to stretch yourself past the set point of feeling just okay, make a commitment to hitting the gym, hiking trail, or yoga studio up to six times a week. (And on the seventh day, rest. We all need rest.)

Self-work is another important aspect of the cross-training program. In life, we are constantly dealing with people and situations that make us feel challenged or uncomfortable, and self-work helps us work through the emotions that come up so that they don't get stuck and poison our field of energy. Not only does self-work keep us from getting bogged down, it actually moves us swiftly along into manifesting more of our potential. Self-work means just that: working on ourselves. It means that we (1) look at where we are, (2) set some goals for where we'd like to be, and then (3) chart the course on how to get there. Here's how my friend Tanya used self-work to get through an obstacle in her life.

Tanya is a forty-two-year-old mother of three who married when she was twenty-five. She was an aerobics instructor when she met her husband, but quit as soon as he got through law school and opened his practice. As the years went by, Tanya stopped exercising and became more involved with her children's school and running the house. When her husband announced he was leaving her, Tanya felt as if she were falling apart. She developed shingles, a painful skin condition brought on by stress, became dependent on antianxiety medications, and was convinced she had cancer because odd little bumps seemed to appear and disappear on her body. Tanya turned to her friends in fury and desperation, bemoaning how badly her husband had treated her by leaving her for another woman. She spent her days telling anyone who would listen how she had been wronged and then settled into each evening with a few glasses of wine and some mind-numbing television.

At this point, I could see that Tanya was not moving forward but was stuck in a holding pattern of feeling sorry for herself. Now, don't get me wrong; she had every reason to be sad and angry, and it's very important that she allowed herself to feel whatever came up. But at a certain point, Tanya had to take charge and begin to address the things in her life that were ailing her. She was not "well" in her body, nor was she thriving emotionally or spiritually. My advice to Tanya was that she begin to do some self-work: if she wanted to grow out of this unpleasant stage, she needed to take responsibility for her life. I told her that once she analyzed the situation and owned up to what part she had played in getting there, she would have the power to start playing differently, and thus create a new reality.

The first thing Tanya had to do was to engage in some self-observation, to ask herself some very important questions:

- What am I feeling right now?

- How familiar is this feeling? Have I, in one way or another, felt it throughout my life?

- Where did these feelings originate?

- What aspect of my psyche is so uncomfortable to look at that it took this situation to force it into my awareness?

- What do I need to do to heal this?

These may seem to be easy enough questions to answer at first glance, but when you are in the middle of a serious interpersonal conflict, health crisis, or even just an ongoing quiet depression, you will see how they lead you right into the wound that needs to be tended to.

We are all wounded in some way. We each have a sacred soft spot, the thing that cuts to the bone and gets our attention and forces us to awaken to our deeper selves. For some it is illness, while for others it is constant drama in our relationships. At various times in our lives, there may be many things we need to work on. But as I see it, the purpose of our lives is to grow and awaken to the powerful potential that is seeded within us, and our most sacred mission is to apply our focus to getting unstuck where we feel stuck.

For Tanya, this meant getting in touch with her anger at being abandoned and tracing it back to being adopted as a baby. As soon as she made the connection, she felt a click of understanding. I advised Tanya that although she couldn't go back and change the past—her birth situation or the split with her husband—she could sit with her pain and apply compassion to the situation. And because it sometimes takes more compassion than we are able to drum up, I guided Tanya to imagine that she could call in the compassion from all the saints and enlightened masters (she is Catholic, so those images worked for her) to flow through her and focus on this part of her wounded self. She could also just imagine that all the love and benevolence in the world was flowing toward and through her, salving the places of pain. Every time she started to nose-dive into that painful place of sorrow and rage, she allowed herself to just feel loved through the discomfort.

After this first step of observation and making the connection, Tanya began to set her goals: She wanted to feel strong and independent, her well-being not contingent on her husband's care and support (or lack thereof). She also wanted to feel energetic when she woke up in the morning, and she wanted that energy to carry her through a purposeful and peaceful day. Tanya wanted a healthy body and a happy outlook. These were big goals and seemingly impossible for someone who had been so mired in stress. But she wrote them down, thought about how they might feel if they manifested themselves, and then she began to chart her course.

At this point, Tanya took up my "throw it all into the pot" approach to wellness. She started praying and meditating, visualizing a life of joy and health. She signed up for a course in restaurant management (she had always loved the fast-paced energy of restaurant kitchens and what happens behind the scenes), and in the meantime secured a job as a hostess at the local hot spot. Tanya also stepped down her antianxiety meds (and wine!) and opted instead to join an anger group so that she could process her feelings with like-minded and healing-oriented peers. The group was free (paid for by donations), so Tanya suffered no financial strain. She also chose to be around healthy, supportive friends who were not likely to allow her to wallow in self-pity. But the most important thing she did was to keep asking herself how she was feeling, and then applying the compassion to the places that hurt. And then she turned toward the proactive steps of creating the life she wanted.

I'm pleased to report that Tanya is happily divorced, dating, financially stable, and as healthy as I've ever seen her.

Self-work can look many different ways to each of us. Sometimes we need contemplation, while at other times we need to invest our energy in taking specific actions. The good results will most likely come from hitting your issue from all angles. Here, then, are the self-work steps to guide your process.

1. **Look at where you are and allow yourself to feel whatever comes up.**
2. **Tend to the places that are wounded.**
3. **Move in the direction of healing by taking pro-active steps.**

Spiritual practice. Regardless of our particular spiritual orientation or religious affiliation, in our self-work we often come around to thinking about our souls and our spirits and what we are (or aren't) doing to nurture them. Spiritual practice reminds us of what's important. Even those of us who would say we are not religious can recognize that we are connected to some sort of deep and unified source, or what I will henceforth refer to as Spirit.

According to Webster's dictionary, the original meaning of worship is "a state or condition of worth." When you embrace worship, then, your aim is to embrace your real worth: the divine perfection that resides within you. No single religion or faith has a patent on this, of course. Whatever spiritual orientation you have, just be sure to build in some time for practice.

In my own life and my work, I have noticed again and again that when we don't have *any* kind of spiritual practice, the ego tends to take over and gets us to thinking of ourselves as separate from the world, disconnected. Spiritual practice brings us back to our identification with something larger. It increases our capacity to love and be kind, both to ourselves and others. At its best, it is directed both inward (learning to love ourselves) and outward (learning to love others). Through spiritual practice—be it regular attendance at a church or a self-styled course of intensive reading in a particular tradition or philosophy—you learn that the more you can transcend the narrow focus of "me and mine," the wider your circle of consideration can become. Thich Nhat Hanh, the Buddhist monk and philosopher, says, "Without a spiritual dimension, we will not have the capacity to confront suffering, to transform suffering and to offer anything to life. A person without a spiritual path is a person walking in darkness. With a path, we are no longer afraid or worried."

There are enough people who live and act in fear that our world is teetering on the brink of enormous change, and as I see it, the goal of any spiritual practice should be to shift the tide for each of us and the world from fear to love, from indifference to compassion. As we nurture the light within us, we can then shine it out onto the world.

As we grow in our faith, even if that just means acknowledging that there is more to life than meets the eye, we find ourselves more comfortable with our power and more directed in our purpose, *and* we are able to count on the support and guidance of a greater intelligence. Having a spiritual practice reminds us of life's important truths: that we are all One, and that what we do to one person or being, we do to ourselves; that all of life is an expression of Spirit; and that at our truest, we are innocent and perfect. Sometimes you need to hear the truth a thousand times or in a thousand different ways before it begins to resonate, but it is still the truth. And putting ourselves in an atmosphere of constant coaching—through attending religious services or reading or praying alone or in a group—increases the velocity of our awakening.

If you do not currently have a spiritual practice, I have a couple of suggestions about choosing a teacher, a philosophy, or a place of worship:

1. **Keep in mind the principles that you want to learn to embody.**
2. **Steer clear of any school of thought that promotes distance, judgment, or ill will.**

Many well-known and established religions have lost the mystical seed embraced by the great wisdom teachings: mercy, forgiveness, humility, benevolence, compassion, selflessness, and integrity. If you do not feel a genuine and widespread love for all people in a particular avenue of practice, consider going elsewhere. According to the system of spiritual development in *A Course in Miracles*, "A church that does not inspire love has a hidden altar that is not serving the purpose for which Spirit intended it."

Keep listening to your inner voice and decide if a teaching appeals to your core goodness or if it resonates with fear-based thinking. There is certainly no need to commit to and stay in one place only; nuggets of wisdom are everywhere you look, so feel free to explore different groups as you gather insights and inspirations.

Service. The eighth pillar is service. It's all too easy to get caught up in life's little dramas and forget about the big picture, but when you reach out and help someone, you feel your sense of purpose and mission kick in. When you give, you strengthen a mind-set of abundance rather than one of lack. Service makes you feel good. It helps you transcend the small self in favor of the higher Self.

Whenever I feel down and think I'm depressed, I ask myself what I've done for someone else lately. Almost every time I get into feeling sorry for myself, I realize that I have been lazy about extending myself for someone else's benefit; I've started to take myself and my everyday agenda way too seriously. Once I dive in to some sort of giving back, I feel useful and grateful that I have something to give. I remember what is important and loosen my grip on the worldly things that had seized my attention. I start feeling more connected and on target, no longer drifting in my self-centered concerns. The blessings I already have in my life become more clear to me, and I stop itching for something that I can never seem to attain.

Years ago I had a client named Jason who seemed to have bad luck at every turn. He was a musician who could not get his music published or played, women didn't give him the time of day, and he seemed to have one malady after another. No matter how hard Jason tried to shift the tide of how his life was playing out, nothing seemed to work. His self-esteem was scraping bottom.

When I asked him if he'd helped anyone out lately, he looked at me like I was crazy. "What do I have to give that anybody would want?" he asked me, in all earnestness.

What I told him, gently and with much encouragement, is that of course he would never know if he never put himself out there! I knew that he'd find something valuable within himself in the act of giving—and that being pulled outside himself would move him out of this stuck place, too.

Jason began teaching music at a juvenile hall. He was shocked to see how many of the kids had never been introduced to musical instruments, much less given the chance to learn how to play them. Even though most of the kids were bouncing off the walls or had serious attitude, a few of them were intrigued by Jason and his instruments. He can pinpoint the exact moment when he looked around at the faces intently watching him and knew he had found his heart's mission.

It didn't take long for me to notice Jason walking taller; he had an air about him that was completely different. His "luck" took a serious turn for the better. He became gainfully employed and met a young woman with whom he felt very connected. His health also improved enormously, perhaps because of some inner strength or reserve that he'd tapped into, or maybe because he now simply cared enough about himself to take better care. The point is, serving others served Jason quite well.

Our culture persuades us to believe that satisfaction will be found in material possessions or powerful positions. We look to bigger houses, better cars, and more impressive friends for our happiness. And no matter how much stuff we accumulate or how far up we get on the corporate ladder, we always want more. That's the way of the ego. But, of course, what we think will make us happy never quite seems to do the trick.

Have you ever wanted something really badly and once you finally owned it or achieved it, you felt let down? It's not only that the getting of something is anticlimactic but also that material things do not hold true value. Being someone's boss or superior is not what the soul craves either. These "wins" appeal to our ego, but not to our Self. When we perceive ourselves as separate (as the ego would have us do) we feel alone and insecure, dwarfed by the vast world "out there." So we grab at what we can, thinking that by attaining things we can at last feel bigger and more secure, more able to stand up to the universe. The ego thinks that if it consumes enough—materially or in the way of position—then it will no longer have anything to fear.

But as you know, all the money in the world doesn't buy you security. The more you get, the more you have to protect. And every time you reach a peak in your job or meet your financial goals, you come across a whole new group of people you have to keep up with or surpass. The ego is like a tapeworm that lives inside you; it always craves more and is never satisfied. You'll never be rich enough or beautiful enough or popular enough or powerful enough to feel *enough* to stand up to the vastness of the universe. When it's you *against* the world instead of you *at one with* the world, things can look pretty daunting. No wonder we feel so anxious!

And so there must be that moment of reckoning when we realize that if we want to be happy, we have to find another way to feel satiated. Instead of looking to the material, we have to look to the ways of Spirit. As soon as you let go of your attachment to the things of this world (and this is a lifelong endeavor, don't worry!), you feel lighter and freer. Your joy comes from giving things away rather than hoarding them. Your power comes from helping others feel better rather than attempting to impose your superiority. You realize that as you serve, so you gain. The great illusion of our ego is that we alone are the center of the universe when, in fact, it is our Oneness— our equality and connectedness with each other—that is the ultimate truth. By doing service, we begin to shift our perspective from the small self to the bigger Self, becoming ever more empathic to the "other"; we realize that this inner change of heart opens us to a broader and more inclusive vision of the world, thus ushering in a more correct relationship with the whole of which we are part.

This insight into our higher potential nourishes the awareness that we are infinitely interconnected with each other and it is in our best interest to "bring up the weakest link" rather than fortify our sole and singular interests. When we realize that overconsuming is not the answer—even more so when our gluttony causes harm to other living creatures and wreaks havoc on our planet—we will want to do everything we can to become more selfless. And so we do service. We help out and volunteer our time, give money, speak up for those who can't speak for themselves, and spread our wealth—in whatever form it takes—around.

When you give from a place of knowing that we are all part of one collective consciousness, you don't pat yourself on the back and say, "I'm so great"; instead you think, "Oh, how lucky I am to have what he needs!" or "Thank goodness I was here just in time to save this poor soul from another day in misery." Another's misery is our misery, because somewhere in the back of our minds, we know it could be us. Or it once was us, or it might one day become us. When we relieve someone else's suffering, we build confidence that should we need it, the world will be there to lift us up.

Remember, we see in the world projections of what is inside us. So if we are generous in our heart, we will see a generous world. If we are loving and compassionate, love and compassion will be reflected back to us. Each of our actions—kind or unkind—ripple out and affect the others around us, and those efforts splash back to us in ways we can't even imagine. When we make another life better, we make our own life better. We are our own—and each other's—savior . . . if we choose to step up to the role. The more you extend yourself in service, the more you will cease feeling alone and insignificant, and you will relax into the awareness that you have become part of the force of evolution and expanding consciousness.

Giving of ourselves makes us feel better in our bodies, too. We feel a rush of euphoria, which is then followed by a sense of calm and fulfillment. This rush is accompanied by a release of endorphins, which provide a sense of emotional well-being. Dr. Wayne Dyer, in his book *The Power of Intention*, points to research that says "a simple act of kindness directed toward another improves the functioning of the immune system and stimulates the production of serotonin in both the recipient of the kindness and the person extending the kindness. Even more amazing is that the persons observing the act of kindness have similar beneficial results." So everyone involved, the giver, the receiver, and the observer are engaged in positive ways when kindness is extended.

Start, if you haven't already, with what you feel most connected to. If you were neglected as a child, for instance, volunteer with kids who have been abused and neglected. If you love animals, work at a rescue shelter or call an animal rights organization to see what you can do to pitch in. If you don't have a lot of time, give money. Certainly, both would be even better! And most of all, stay involved with local and national politics. Look closely at what your representatives are doing and what the overall and long-term effects are. Study the issues and let them know what you think. It's amazing what one person can do when they set their mind to it. We can make this world kinder; we just have to keep our heart open and stay active and generous. When we demonstrate love or compassion or concern, we are walking in the footsteps of spiritual giants; we are fulfilling our highest potential as human beings.

These various tools and practices will pop up throughout the book. As you encounter areas where you're stuck or feel particularly challenged, turn back to this chapter and try a few of the tools from this cross-training tool kit and see if they don't lead you back in the direction of your own health and happiness. And remember, once you set your intention in a given direction, life has a way of getting you there.

PART TWO

Clearing the Way

CHAPTER THREE

Shine a Little Light
Transforming the Shadow

SOCRATES FAMOUSLY STATED THAT "THE UNEXAMINED LIFE IS NOT worth living." Many great thinkers and writers have written about the tendency of human beings to live a sort of autopilot existence, moving from activity to activity, doing what comes next without thinking much about it or feeling any sort of transcendent power. Virginia Woolf wrote touchingly of those "moments of being" when we move outside of reaction in our lives and into action, when we are fully present to the world around us, and make conscious choices rather than unconscious ones. Awakening and evolving and enjoying our lives fully is first and foremost a matter of knowing ourselves and what makes us feel most alive.

An important task on this path of wellness is going to be looking at some of the blockages—in our bodies and emotions—that are keeping us in pain or feeling stuck. From the time we are children, if we are to survive, we learn to mask some of our more difficult feelings. We have to. We learn quickly that it isn't safe to be angry about having to put down our book to come to the dinner table or to be sad that Mommy or Daddy seems too distracted to listen to another story. Getting angry or feeling sad makes Mommy raise her voice or Daddy leave the house. We learn to push away challenging or uncomfortable feelings. Fortunately, we humans are survivors, and denial and re-pression are some of the best defenses in our arsenal. Trouble is, re-pressed emotions get stuck in our bodies and our fields of energy, causing anxiety, depression, and a whole host of other physical man-ifestations such as heartburn, stiff neck, or worse.

Ironically, perhaps, repressed (denied) feelings don't ever dis-appear; in fact, they do the opposite. The more we try *not* to feel some-thing, the more life seems to supply events that will trigger the exact emotion we don't want. This may indeed be our own inner wisdom pulling us forward in our evolution by attracting exactly those situa-tions that will make us face the repressed feelings head on.

If you aren't comfortable with anger, for instance, life will tend to keep on giving you reasons to be angry until you are forced to fi-nally look squarely at your anger and deal with it. No matter how many times you tell yourself to "rise above it" or "let it go," situa-tions will keep presenting themselves that will make it very difficult for you to do anything *but* experience the avoided emotion. You can continue to feel like a "victim" or take a good and honest look at what part you are playing. Until we realize that what we see outside us is somehow also inside us, we are powerless to change it.

I have had many clients who swear they aren't angry, but, for rea-sons that are vexing to them, they experience an unusual abundance of betrayals or slights. As each betrayal seems more egregious than the last, they have to work harder and harder at "not being angry." When it finally gets to be too much and they consider the possibil-ity that maybe, just maybe, there is something they are not conscious of, then the work of healing can begin.

Take my client Lori, for example. Lori is a fortyish real estate broker who used to be an actress. She had gotten a few small parts throughout her career, usually as an "extra" or stand-in. When she switched careers to start selling houses, she said she knew that "it was the universe calling her to do something that had more of a future, less rejection." When her on-again, off-again boyfriend of six years finally called it quits for good, Lori said she was grateful that he ended what she would never have been able to. Even though he was not kind to her, she had put up with all his misbehavior because they had shared some chemistry that she couldn't turn away from. When she was diagnosed with cancer, Lori resigned herself to the belief that she was just unlucky and had to play the lousy cards she'd been dealt with as much dignity as possible. And when the neighbor next door started doing construction just as she began chemotherapy, she moved to the other side of the house in order to avoid the earsplitting noise.

At none of these points did Lori even consider that she might have the right and a reason to be angry. Enraged, even. When she was little, Lori's parents had scolded her on several occasions for speaking out against them, telling her, "You should be ashamed of yourself. Good girls don't get angry. Look at yourself in the mirror: Who would ever want to be near such an ugly face all grimaced in anger?" So she learned not to be angry. The problem was, of course, that she *was* angry. And for good reason.

Lori had long forgotten what it felt like just to allow an emotion to come up and flow through her. I suggested to her that life kept lobbing more and more things at her to be angry about until she was finally forced to just go ahead and feel that very thing she was shamed out of feeling all those years before. I explained that she didn't have to take her anger out on anyone (scream at her acting agent for not getting her work or fight with her ex-boyfriend until he saw that he had wronged her or knock at the neighbors' door like a lunatic until they halted the noise); *she just had to allow herself to feel it.* And by simply getting in touch with her anger, life would most probably back off on what seemed to be an assault on her patience.

Our goal as holistically well human beings is to become fully integrated with all the different parts of ourselves, to learn to love all of it. Even the so-called dark or "ugly" parts. And as we learn to accept and love ourselves, our energy lightens up, life gets easier, and we contribute to an awakened and aware world.

I coached Lori to work out on a boxing bag, scream at the top of her lungs in a closed car where no one could hear her, and practice writing some wicked letters she would never send. This way, she didn't hurt anyone with her emotion, but neither did she keep it bottled up inside, ashamed at the magnitude of what she was feeling. Lori no longer makes excuses when things don't work out favorably; she breathes into the anger and processes it responsibly. She is a whole lot healthier and happier since she has started this awareness practice.

As we drop into the feelings we were afraid of and explore them, we will find that life oddly seems to throw us far fewer agitations. I venture that the very purpose of the agitations, from a metaphysical point of view, is to get our attention, to get us thinking about what we need to address. And once the healing process sets in, the agitations become unnecessary. Once the repressed emotion has been attended to—responsibly processed and released—it is thus disempowered. And then things seem to "magically" get better all around. Of course, this requires practice.

There are many tools that can help you come face-to-face with your feelings, and you've probably tried some of them. Journaling, self-help books, meditation, body work—they all can help you get in touch with and release bottled-up emotions. But you can't release what you don't even see. If you can't get in touch with these feelings on your own, a good therapist or counselor can lead you through the walls of denial and resistance. The kind of therapy you choose doesn't necessarily matter. What matters is that you trust and respect the person and have a good relationship with her or him.

The very act of opening up and sharing your story is what initiates the process of healing. By having a responsible and caring person listen with attention and compassion to your story, you will feel heard and validated. As we discussed earlier, this kind of deep self-work doesn't have to cost a lot of money, but it does take your commitment. Twelve-step groups are a great resource for fellowship, as are myriad support groups for whatever problem you may be delving into. Many religious institutions have counselors available, and there are clinics that scale their fees for people who cannot afford therapy. Lectures, workshops, and retreats are also wonderful, as is, of course, a good and trusted friend.

We all need to be witnessed; we need to know that what we feel makes sense in some way. Once the memory or secret comes to light, a therapist or support person can help you retrain your behavior in the areas in which you had an exaggerated or inappropriate emotional response. If you are working alone on this, talk out loud. Let your voice be heard even when you're just by yourself. Any way that you can move the energy from being stuck inside is helpful. Your relationships will get better, your body will no longer hold the cellular memories of pain or unresolved business, and you will have a greater sense of freedom and happiness.

But our emotions are also affected by the way we treat our bodies. Surely you have experienced a "sugar low" when you have been bingeing on snacks or desserts; you feel edgy and tired until you get a fix. In this case, there are concrete physiological influences that are affecting your emotions. The body, mind, and spirit are always engaged in a dance. There is no separation between them.

If we want to transform ourselves into happier, healthier people, we have to be willing to look at all the factors that affect our well-being. If you're tired, in other words, it's important to ask yourself not only whether you are eating correctly or getting enough sleep, but also if you have some issue that is weighing you down inside and robbing you of vitality. The integrative approach has us looking, always, at all aspects of the situation.

As you begin to look deeply at your health and well-being, you will realize that few symptoms have just one cause or dimension. For instance, if you have a pain in your lower back, it might very well be that you slept on your pillows wrong and simply need a massage or chiropractic adjustment. If the pain has been going on for a long time, you may have seen a physical therapist, gotten an MRI, or possibly considered surgery. From an integrative perspective, however, that pain, real as it is, might also point to a deeply held unexpressed or unrealized emotion.

How Emotions "Cause" Physical Pain

Dr. John Sarno, a world-renowned specialist in pain and mind-body disorders, says that a great number of patients with back or neck pain—or even allergies, acid reflux, or irritable bowel syndrome— have unknowingly created the malady themselves in order to keep their conscious awareness away from an unpleasant emotion that threatens their comfort zone. According to Sarno, the emotion we are most averse to is rage, anger that has gathered steam from being kept down and locked away.

A lot of people who think of themselves as good people—Sarno calls them "goodists," because they tend to be very much tied to an image of themselves as nice and good people—do not at all feel comfortable with such a "distasteful" and potentially out-of-control emotion as rage. If something happens in their life that sparks intense anger, these people tend not to deal with it, because they don't like what it brings up in them. Say the boss is being unfair or work conditions are overwhelming. A goodist might well submerge his true feelings because he doesn't want to rock the boat. He convinces himself that he has "let it go," when, in fact, by not allowing himself to experience his authentic emotions, they have just gone unconscious.

When we don't think we can handle something in a way that feels safe and manageable—i.e., if we speak up, we might lose a relationship or job or, even worse, be thought of as a bad person—our survival mechanism kicks in and buries the feelings in the recesses of our psyche. Those disowned feelings become part of our shadow.

Carl Jung described the shadow as our dark side, the unconscious part of us that houses all the raw thoughts and desires we are ashamed to admit to. This part of our psyche contains those aspects of our character that—because of a disapproving society, shaming parent, or strict religious ethos—we cannot acknowledge or act out. Because when we were very young we received the message that these traits were bad, we repressed or denied them. To our conscious mind, these inadmissible parts of our self ceased to exist. In their place we developed a mask, a more pleasing and acceptable front to present to the world. We committed to being "good" and kept tucked away what we were taught was "bad."

This vision of who we should and shouldn't be is deeply ingrained in us and is part of our identity, and so we strongly reject any feeling or awareness that threatens it. So when the shadow tries to make itself known, when the repugnant and disclaimed anger or sadness starts to arise in our conscious awareness, our instinct for survival kicks into high gear and creates a powerful distraction. That distraction looks like an infection, an ache, or any malady that is distinct and bothersome enough to get our attention. This is what is called a psychosomatic condition. The pain or illness is *absolutely real*, but its origin is emotional or mental.

As Dr. Sarno puts it, the brain is in cahoots with the body in such a way that when the repulsive emotion starts to come up, the body will quickly conjure an intense localized pain or discomfort that is big enough to make us forget what we were beginning to feel. Basically, the brain says, "Whoa! I can't let myself feel that rage. It threatens my identity as a good and nice person. Good and nice people do not have rage; it is unseemly and out of control. I will send a signal to the tendons and muscles in a certain section of my lower back so that it seizes up with pain, and then I will completely forget about that nasty emotion because I will be too busy focusing on how much my back hurts and what I can do to make it stop."

Sound incredible? Well, of course none of this is done consciously. We don't realize what's happening; all we know is that our lower back is hurting and we want the pain to go away. We obsess about what could have caused it and what we can do to cure it. That obsession keeps us from thinking about the emotion that was just about to emerge into our conscious awareness. And voila! What was disowned and rejected—most likely rage—is shoved down once again, deep within the shadowy part of the psyche.

How does the mind-body pull off this trick? What is the physiological mechanism that allows this to take place?

The brain simply orders a reduction of blood flow to a certain area, depriving it of oxygen, which results in pain. Dr. Sarno points out that chronic pain shows up in an area that makes sense in your life. Our bodies/brains are very clever that way. For instance, a tennis player might develop tennis elbow. He wouldn't tend to look too deeply for an explanation, as he would if the pain or affliction had seemed to come out of nowhere. The fact that it "makes sense" further protects us from the scary emotion.

Here's another way this psychosomatic pain tends to "make sense," thus keeping us from looking at it too closely: Let's say you know a lot of people who have sinus infections. As you are about to get close to an old, complicated emotion, you might suddenly develop a psychosomatic sinus infection, because your conscious mind would be satisfied that sinus infections are common and therefore not worth investigating on an emotional level. "Ah, yes. I have a terrible sinus infection. They seem to be going around these days and I hear that they are very difficult to treat. I must figure out what the best protocol is for this. I must call so-and-so for the name of his doctor so I can figure out how to beat this thing."

And so the obsession with the difficult malady begins. No room to think about feelings. The foil worked, and for the moment you didn't have to think about the internal and unresolved issues or feelings that were starting to emerge.

By the way, difficult feelings often begin to emerge when we are quiet; when we go on vacation or are enjoying a weekend of rest. The shadow sees an opening and goes for it.

Even when you treat the symptom with surgery or medication and it seems to go away, in most cases, the symptom will either come back or the mind-body will invent a new problem to claim your attention. In fact, the psyche will often find something equal or more powerful in its attention-getting ability to replace the old complaint. You can "cure" the presenting malady, but if you still have a powerful disowned emotion lurking beneath the surface, some other symptom or ache will arise to take its place.

How brilliantly the mind and body work together to save us from disturbing experiences!

You see, growth is often uncomfortable. The shadow becomes the shadow because we don't want to deal with what it represents. We don't want to see ourselves in a certain light, so we tuck away what we think is repulsive or frightening or disagreeable. But because our nature is to evolve and become ever more enlightened, the part of us that is dark will constantly try to come to light. That disowned part of us wants to be heard and accepted.

The emotions we are afraid of are the very things we have to come to terms with if we are to move forward. Picture your shadow as a rejected little bully of a kid; the more you try to dismiss the scruffy little fellow, the more feisty he becomes in getting in your face. He only wants love; he only wants to be accepted and invited into the light of day. If you don't willingly invite him into the light of your awareness (integrate him), he will get your attention some other way. He will force you to reckon with him.

Unfinished business does not go away; it only gets louder and more pressing. It will keep repeating itself until we pay attention and process what needs to be heard and accepted. If we are resistant to our anger, the world will give us reasons to be angry. If we are repulsed by our feelings of weakness or sadness, the world will rain down on us reasons to be sad until we crack open and feel the sadness. What we resist persists.

Facing Our Demons

Alas, we are meant to crack open so that we become deeper, more compassionate, and more evolved human beings.

As children we didn't have the tools to deal with certain difficult emotions, but as adults we have to carefully open ourselves up to the feelings or issues that scare us. We can only begin to truly heal by connecting to the disowned feelings and letting them be expressed. We can scream in a closed car, beat a pillow, or curl into a ball and cry for hours. None of this will kill us; it will in fact heal us.

Please don't misunderstand. If you are experiencing physical pain or symptoms of a serious disease, by all means take it seriously and see a professional who can help you. Just consider that very often there is an emotional component to chronic pain or debility, and to the extent that you can address the issue in a holistic way, you will heal and move forward along your wellness continuum in a more robust way.

Once we make peace with our demons—be they rage or fear or shame, and we all have them—we become more fully integrated human beings. You see, a person who is in touch with her feelings does not need to manifest symptoms physically because she is already paying attention to what is going on inside.

So next time you experience pain that won't go away or some illness that keeps plaguing you, remember that many health issues arise to get our attention. Ask yourself what feelings or memories you might be trying to avoid. Know that if something is unconscious, it means you truly do not know it's there. It is certainly not your fault or a sign of weakness! But by developing a curiosity, a willingness to investigate, you dramatically increase your chances of healing.

When you go about this process of allowing your emotions without judgment, you will be led into your Truth. Ask yourself if there is anger—rage even—that you need to connect with and then heal. Allow yourself to drop into deep sadness or grief even if your normal instinct is to pull yourself up by the bootstraps and "get over it." Even if you might be tempted to think that some things would be better off left alone, look into them anyway. As Jesus is quoted as saying in the Gospel of Thomas, "If you bring forth that which is within you, what you bring forth will save you. If you do not bring forth what is within you, what you do not bring forth will destroy you."

Exercise: Owning Your Full Range of Feelings

Here are a few questions to ask yourself should you be experiencing pain or discomfort, either physically or emotionally:

- If I get very quiet and listen, is there a hidden or disowned feeling(s) that is trying to become known?

- When did I first experience this feeling? Did I have this feeling in childhood? What brought it on?

- How does this feel historical? In other words, does this situation fit a pattern?

- Why do I not allow myself just to have this feeling? What am I afraid of?

- Could I simply allow myself to have the feeling without acting it out in a destructive manner?

- What could I do to process this feeling without hurting anyone, including myself?

- After processing it responsibly, could I let it go?

At the risk of repeating myself, I'll tell you this: feelings don't just go away when you ignore them. They just work harder to get your attention. They pop up in inappropriate ways (you blow your top at someone who doesn't really deserve it, for example) and often manifest physically (heartburn, headaches, anxiety attacks, or worse) until you finally sit down and look within to see what is trying to be healed. Your shadow is not an enemy; it is a part of you and it is what makes you human. To be fully integrated and well, get to know your shadow. Coax it out and listen to it. You will grow to know yourself better, and thus intuit the steps you must take in order to keep progressing.

It's easy to feel overwhelmed by the prospect of having to look at every ailment multidimensionally. How will you ever know if you've gotten to the *real* roots of it? Fortunately, the body, mind, and spirit ask only that you approach your illness from an integrative perspective and adopt an attitude of curiosity about it. If you do these things, chances are you *will* get to the core problem and deal with it, thus bringing yourself to a higher level of wellness.

Try this:

1. Try to become aware of the emotions that lie beneath the surface of your physical discomfort. Disowned emotions can show up in the body as pain or illness, and in order to heal and become healthfully integrated we have to deal with this emotional material as well.

2. Approach whatever troubles you from each of the angles of body, mind, and spirit. Look for the physical causes as well as the emotional and spiritual ones. A complete and well-rounded understanding of the causation is imperative.

3. Sit quietly and ask yourself a few leading questions. This will often bring you to your emotions. If you feel stuck, or overwhelmed, seek the help of a therapist or counselor.

CHAPTER FOUR

How to Hear Yourself Think
Clearing Mental Chatter

JUST AS IMPORTANT AS GETTING TO OUR CORE EMOTIONS IS THE WORK OF quieting our minds so we can hear what our soul is trying to tell us. Our minds can cause all kinds of chaos and confusion in our bodies and threaten our sense of equanimity and peace. That's because the mind is constantly at work processing past events and setting us up for what happens next. It is full to bursting with preconceptions, anxieties, and old agendas that we might not even be aware of. It's time to get quiet and find out. By clearing out all that mental clutter, we can finally hear what really matters to us. And set our lives going in that direction.

In this chapter we'll look at a few exercises that are highly informative in this regard.

Exercise: Stream of Consciousness

The closest thing we have to a tool for hearing our own thoughts and thought process is journaling or talking into a tape recorder. Recording your mental chatter or stream of consciousness is like taking a snapshot of your own mind.

For this exercise, set your watch—or timer—for twenty minutes: this will prevent you from being concerned about time restraints.

Now, just record every thought that passes through your mind. It's of the utmost importance that you don't judge or edit yourself in this process. Know that there are no good or bad, right or wrong thoughts. Thoughts are merely energies passing in and out of existence; they come and go. Simply let your inner voices be heard as you record them.

Next, review where your mind went in those twenty minutes. What kind of thoughts ran through your consciousness? What sort of images were consistently present? Was there anger? Worry? Joy? Excitement? As you identify the emotions that came up for you, notice how your mind builds stories around them. When I first did this exercise, I noticed myself worrying about things that I had yet to get done. I had a lot of "busy-ness" thoughts that created anxiety for me. When I followed that train of thought, I noticed that the feeling that came up right behind my to-do list was that I would never be good enough or get enough done to feel okay and worthwhile. I felt a desperation to be accepted and appreciated, and most of that desire to get things accomplished—both small and significant—was about my insecurity. Quite an insight to work with!

The mind can be a master manipulator; and just as you would with a manipulative person, it's essential to identify the mind's techniques. For example, when she was trying to break free from an addiction to high-fat sweets, a client confided in me that her mind took her on the same type of journey nearly every time. It began in a positive way, with the exercise of self-control, but then she veered toward the familiar old ways of indulging. It went something like this: "I'm not going to eat that pint of ice cream. Mmm, but it looks so good. Maybe this could be the last time. Well, if this is really going to be the last time, I should go ahead and treat myself because I'm never going to eat ice cream again. I'll have a big bowlful and then that's it." She took this journey with her mind time and time again as she tried to quit her ice cream habit.

Finally, she realized her own self-sabotage and was able to come to terms with her thought process in a whole new way. She realized that she could have those very thoughts but then redirect them. She could reframe her craving by finding something else "sweet and delicious" but better for her. Rather than trying to "quit" sweets for good, for instance, she could begin eating an individual square of really good dark chocolate along with a cup of green tea (both are high in antioxidants, which are widely considered to be protective from heart disease, lung cancer, prostate cancer, asthma, and type 2 diabetes). Instead of her mind using her, she could learn to use her mind.

You can strengthen your will and mind through an awareness of your thought process, and this strength can assist you in overcoming great obstacles and achieving even greater dreams. Abstaining from high-fat sweets is a very clear, concrete example, but now you can look at what kind of process leads you into indulgence in heartache, despair, anger, or anything self-destructive. These states are just as real, and in most cases, more undesirable than an addiction to ice cream, if they are recurring and damaging problems. The trick is to listen to the voice that presents itself, develop an understanding and compassion for how it got there, and then logically lead yourself into new thought territory.

Exercise: Three Days of Journaling

If the journaling or recording exercise worked for you, try doing it for three days in a row. Every day, journal a few times throughout the day, writing down whatever arises. Get in touch with how your mind is working. Try not to judge your mind or yourself; this exercise is about becoming aware of your process, and honesty is essential. During these three days, don't try to implement any changes. This is a time of insight that will ultimately (and with hardly any effort) bring about the upgrade you seek.

At the end of every day, review your journal entry. Use a high-lighter to mark repetitive thoughts, patterns, or stories. Note any events in your life that you review again and again, harping on wrongs, mistakes, or missed opportunities. Identify the personal stories that your mind likes to tell you again and again. Perhaps you'll notice the same thought recurring, but with different names, faces, or locations. Highlight these as well.

On the fourth day, begin to do a mental housecleaning. Determine which of your stories, thoughts, and mental habits are no longer helpful. For example, you may have noticed in your journaling exercise that you tend to be hard on yourself throughout the day. Perhaps you locked your keys in the car, and your mental process went something like this, "Look what I did. I'm so stupid. How could I do that? What an idiot I am." What good does that kind of mental berating do anyone? Perhaps you'd like to replace that process with this one: "Aha. I have locked the keys in the car. Oh, look how tempted I am to berate myself . . . but no! I am quite a smart person with perhaps too much on my plate. Maybe I need to slow down and give myself a few moments throughout the day to simply rest and regenerate. I see that I am really pushing myself to get so much done just so that I can feel I'm pulling my weight. Keys locked in the car is not such a big deal; but appreciating myself for who I am—whether I get it all done or not—*is* a big deal. What a great little learning opportunity this has been. I'm actually glad this happened, because it called attention to some negative self-talk I need to rework."

This is a quantum shift in attitude. Addressing your self-loathing is the most profound work you can do, because as you learn to accept and love yourself for all your so-called foibles, you will become a kinder and more peaceful person, which will not only make you more well, but will make the world just that much more friendly.

As you find mental patterns that need to be healed or upgraded, it is also essential that you take note of what *is* working up there in that brain of yours. So give yourself credit when you notice you are thinking thoughts that are joyful, kind, and creative. Be grateful for how evolved you already are!

Try this:

1. **Break negative thought habits simply by noticing them and then reframing them more positively.**

2. **Curb thoughts of self-loathing as they come up. Simply catch yourself having the thought and then decide to be more loving. This will not only make you feel better and happier, it will also add to the world being a kinder and more peaceful place.**

3. **Make journaling a habit. It's one of the best and simplest ways of keeping in touch with how you really feel.**

CHAPTER FIVE

A Jump Start for Your Body
Doing a Cleanse

OF COURSE THE BEDROCK OF WELLNESS IS FEELING GOOD IN YOUR BODY
and being aware of what helps and hurts it, and one of the best ways
I know to jump-start the process of feeling good in your body is
through a body cleanse.

A cleanse is a short-term fast, during which you give up certain
foods (or sometimes all food) for a period of time. People tend to
think of cleansing and fasting as difficult and exotic Eastern practices undertaken by monks or political heroes like the liberation
leader of India, Mahatma Gandhi. In fact, the founders of Western
medicine as we know it today, Hippocrates, Galen, and Paracelsus,
prescribed cleansing and fasting as a means of preventing and even
curing disease. Paracelsus wrote, "Fasting is the greatest remedy, the
physician within." It has been a staple of good health throughout history: even the giants of Western intellectual development, Plato,
Socrates, and Pythagoras, practiced regular fasting, and required it
of their students as well. Plutarch, the Greek philosopher, wrote, "Instead of using medicine, rather fast a day." Giving up the comfort of
certain foods is a tried-and-true means of enhancing, preserving, and
enlivening physical as well as spiritual well-being. It's not just good
for the body, it's also a very important part of a general clearing and

lightening that can have a considerable effect on our moods, our outlook, and our sense of spiritual connectedness. Again, this is all about body, mind, and spirit. They rarely act or react alone.

If you have never done a cleanse before, this may sound a bit daunting. I completely understand. It's always challenging to put the brakes on what feels comfortable, especially in so elemental an area as eating. But any time you disrupt a pattern or meet a challenge, you create an enormous space for a quantum leap to happen. You clear the way for new energy and new awarenesses to come in.

What are some more good reasons for doing a cleanse?

It takes a lot of work to break down food, keep all the organs and systems running, and deal with stress. The body doesn't have the luxury of putting everything else on hold so that it can tend to the deeper issues of processing and releasing the stored toxins, extra fat, and waste that have accumulated over the years. When you put certain foods on the back burner for a bit, your body has a reprieve from its normal everyday chore of digesting difficult things, and it can really dig into that much-needed heavier work.

Even as our bodies are uniquely designed to survive under less-than-ideal conditions, we still need to take proactive steps to maximize our ability to heal, regenerate, and operate at optimal capacity. When the body is overburdened with too many toxins, it simply isn't able to function efficiently and, over time, we will feel "off our game" and perhaps get sick.

Many toxins find their way into the human body and we have very few means of getting rid of them short of a cleanse. When you cleanse, you create a break in the workload so that the body's innate wisdom can tend to some of the old stored-up junk. Artificial flavors, synthetic coloring agents, pesticides, herbicides, fungicides, and insecticides are just a few of the many toxins regularly consumed by the average person. These chemicals are often stored in fatty and other tissues in the body, and build up over time. Add in environmental pollution and complex medications and you have a brilliant recipe for the impairment of optimal bodily function.

Those who cleanse their bodies regularly (one to three times per year) report increased energy, enhanced immune function, fewer cravings for unhealthy, junky foods, greater mental clarity and acuity, clearer skin, fresher breath, brighter eyes, and an enhanced sense of well-being. The body knows how to heal if we give it the opportunity; we just need to stop piling on the extra burdens for a bit so that it can work its magic.

Remember that a cleanse is only temporary; it is a short-term vacation for your body, giving it time to rest and detox. No one's asking you to give up anything forever, unless of course you discover that you want to. Just try to stay open and willing to go the distance. And remember that everything is connected, so as you take care of your body through this cleanse, your mental and spiritual health will also improve, thereby upgrading your relationships, your work, and every other aspect of your life.

Step 1. Take Note and Learn: Keep an Inventory

Before starting your cleanse, take a few days and become more aware of your current eating patterns. For three days, keep an inventory of everything you put into your body. Note the time, how much you eat or drink, and what your mood was as you consumed. Becoming aware of *how you feel while you eat* is an essential piece of the health puzzle, especially for emotional eaters. You may notice that when you feel sad, you tend to eat—or overeat—carbohydrates. Many people turn to sugar or caffeine when they are tired. Others go to fats when they feel anxiety. Once you start looking at how and why you eat the way you do, you may find that you use food to self-medicate (take yourself out of an uncomfortable emotional state) rather than just to nourish the body with what it actually wants or needs. We all do this to some extent, but the trick is to gradually become more conscious of our inner workings. Remember, you can't change anything until you first have awareness; when something is unconscious, it cannot be shifted or changed because you don't even realize it's there. So be vigilant in your observations and write down everything you ingest and why.

After three days of taking an inventory of your eating and drinking behaviors, look over your notes. First, notice how you feel about your eating patterns. Do you feel proud and happy with what you have chosen to put in your body? Or are you more embarrassed or worried? Where do you see room for improvement? Are there addictive qualities to your eating that might be damaging to your health? Does it seem like you eat too much of one type of food and not enough of another? Write down all your observations with as much objectivity as possible.

When I did this, I couldn't believe how many sweets I was consuming. I used to have at least two desserts a day (one after lunch and one after dinner), something sweet and bready for breakfast, and a juice (which I thought was healthy but have since realized is loaded with sugar, naturally occurring or not) somewhere in between. I saw so clearly what a sweet tooth I had and that it had taken me and my physiology hostage. But as I looked closer, I saw that those sweets were ways of comforting myself when I felt empty or lonely. I literally felt like I went into some sort of a trance as I ate my desserts; I don't even think I fully tasted them. I just knew that for a few minutes, I wasn't feeling a gnawing sadness that I didn't want to address.

I also noticed that the more sweet stuff I ate, the more I wanted. I saw that I slipped into this cycle of blood-sugar highs and lows and it became an enormous distraction for me to try to control and manage the peaks and valleys. Because I was struggling with trying to get a handle on my diet and ballooning stomach, I didn't have time to deal with things in my life that were making me sad. Convenient.

Step 2. Set an Intention

After becoming aware and alert to our inner workings and patterns of behavior, we can set our intentions for any changes we'd like to make in regard to eating and drinking. Perhaps you would like to eat more slowly or sit at a table. Or eat at least one whole fruit and three servings of fresh organic vegetables a day. Or say grace before digging in.

After my first cleanse, I decided that I didn't want to talk during breakfast but preferred to eat quietly, by myself, as the morning broke. I also resolved to at least have sweets that have a lower glycemic index (foods that don't spike your blood sugar), since I wasn't ready to give up the taste altogether. I would switch from caramels to bittersweet chocolate. And I would have cookies sweetened with agave nectar or brown-rice syrup rather than white sugar.

My intention was to phase out the sugar frenzies by gently easing off the hard-core desserts and choosing health food versions instead. Something that helped me with my craving for sweets is a supplement called Nopal Cactus that is reputed to even out your blood sugar so that you aren't swinging from high to low and grabbing the next sugary treat to fulfill the insane craving. I also started drinking a "green drink"—a powdered mix of wheatgrass and various other vegetables—at around four PM, when my energy usually dipped.

By taking these little steps, I eased myself out of some habits that were steering my health into a bad place. My intention was to eat healthfully without feeling deprived and to enjoy an abundance of energy.

So, as you set your intentions, consider what kinds of foods are harmonious with your beliefs and knowledge of health, and then set your sights on working them into your plan. Then rehearse in your mind what it would feel like if you ate and drank like a healthy, conscious person. Visualize yourself sitting down to your ideal table with the ideal meal in front of you. Feel the feelings you would like to have while eating. As you imagine it, add in as much detail as you possibly can so that your mind and body become attuned to a heightened way of being. And as is the key to all effective visualization, feel the gratitude for this wonderful experience that is being seeded in your mind. You are training your energy to become healthy and conscious.

Step 3. Start Cleansing!

Every individual has different needs, as dictated by your past medical history and medications, so it's important not to begin this or any significant change to your diet without first consulting your doctor. Choose a doctor, if you can, who is well versed in integrative medicine (medicine that combines allopathic care with alternative and natural approaches) so that you have the most up-to-date and well-rounded advice.

This Jump-Start Cleanse will eliminate sources of toxins and allergens, giving the digestive system a break from working overtime to process the substances that inhibit optimum performance the most. Again, increased energy, better digestion, and relief from various aches and pains (including headaches, muscle aches, and joint pain) are just a few of the known benefits. As with each of the practices in this book, this cleanse, which you might think of as something you do for your physical body, has its emotional and spiritual components as well. As you eliminate sugar, for instance, you might experience the feelings you were unconsciously trying to escape by indulging in desserts. Since you no longer have the distraction of the whole cycle of craving a sweet—trying to resist eating it, indulging anyway, and then feeling guilty about it—you are left simply with that *feeling* you had been trying to avoid. Which might be uncomfortable, yes, but as discussed earlier, awareness is good. Being in touch with our feelings, even if they aren't "pleasant," is key to our ultimate well-being.

And on a spiritual level, when I first did a cleanse, I couldn't believe how difficult it was for me to give up the foods I had become attached to, even knowing that the cleanse would only last a couple of weeks. It became clear how enslaved I was by my habits inasmuch as my mood was ruled by my ability to eat the goodies that I loved and was used to. I realized that if I was to be on a serious spiritual path, I had to look at all my attachments, including food habituations. If I was to continue growing and evolving, I had to be able to see where I was not free. The cleanse helped me to identify some glitches where I was *not* able to choose out of freedom rather than habit, and so I was able to focus more effort on becoming more conscious.

Stay on this program for as many days as you can, up to twenty-one days, as your ambition, willingness, and ability allow. Just do the best you can and don't worry about perfection. The first time around, you may go just a day or two. That's fine. Just give it a try. Take one day at a time. Don't look too far ahead. Who knows? You may surprise yourself when you find yourself on day fourteen!

For the next several days, up to twenty-one, please avoid the following:

- **sugar**
- **alcohol**
- **caffeine**
- **gluten**
- **animal products**

Why? Let's take each one in turn.

Sugar. When you eat sugar, it turns into glucose in your blood. When your body notices that your glucose levels are high, in other words that there is more sugar in your system than you need at the moment, it produces insulin in the pancreas. Insulin, in turn, is released into the body to store the glucose that is sitting in your blood not being burned up. The more sugar, or glucose, you take in, the more insulin your body will produce and release. Insulin stores the glucose in the form of glycogen in your liver and muscles, and when that limited storage space is full, insulin will help turn the sugar energy into fat.

Unfortunately for sugar lovers, insulin can have harmful effects, and your cells know this. It can inflame all the cells it comes into contact with. This inflammation is not only the beginning of the fatal cellular breakdown known as aging, but also the inflammatory conditions associated with it, including cancer and other degenerative illnesses.

In fact, past and current studies around the world have demonstrated a connection between sugar (and other foods that register in the body with a high glycemic index, like white flour and processed starches) and cancer. A collaborative study conducted at the Harvard School of Public Health reports that "a diet high in glycemic load may increase the risk of pancreatic cancer in women who already have an underlying degree of insulin resistance." Normally, insulin escorts glucose from the bloodstream into the cells of the body, not unlike a key opening a door. In some people, the cells of the body are resistant to insulin's action. It is as if their cells have "locks" that are clogged with chewing gum and no longer respond to the insulin "key." The Department of Oncological Sciences at the University of Utah found similar results in their study of colon cancer, stating, "These findings support previous reports that dietary sugars, especially a diet high in simple carbohydrates, increase the risk of colon cancer." Scientists at the Universities of Toronto and Milan in collaboration with the International Agency for Research on Cancer in Lyon, France, have shown "moderate direct associations between glycemic index or glycemic load and breast cancer risk, and consequently, a possible role of insulin resistance in breast cancer development." Ovarian cancer associations with sugar consumption have been reported by the *International Journal of Cancer*.

Sugar is physically addictive. It causes your energy receptors to become overwrought, and in a sense, deadened, so that you may not feel energized by anything but sugar. If you're eating too much sugar, you may feel lethargic and slow after consuming other foods, a low that makes your physical craving for the pick-me-up of sugar even more intense. This is how a physical addiction operates. You experience a roller coaster ride of energetic ups and downs, with the lows slowly growing longer, and the highs shrinking steadily, until the consumption of sugar brings on only fatigue, as does the consumption of any other food. When this occurs, know that you're likely well on your way to type 2 diabetes, a condition in which your body can no longer process the massive amounts of toxic, inflammatory insulin it is producing in its vain attempt to protect you from sugar.

In addition, digesting any amount of sugar leaches the body of essential vitamins and upsets the balance of minerals, which could lead to copper and chromium deficiencies and inhibit the absorption of magnesium and calcium. Sugar contributes to obesity in both children and adults. It increases the risk of heart disease in some people by raising triglycerides (the form in which fat is carried by the blood). In excess, sugar can be converted to fat, and is carried in the bloodstream in particles called triglycerides. This tends not to happen when people have healthier carbohydrates—fruits, vegetables, beans, and whole grains. This is important, because triglycerides can contribute to heart disease, in much the same way as cholesterol does.

It creates an ideal environment for systemic infections and tooth loss, preceded by tooth decay and periodontal disease. Absentmindedness, poor long- and short-term memory, learning disorders, erratic, disruptive behavior, difficulty concentrating, and the impediment of the learning capability of the brain in both adults and children can be caused by the consumption of sugar. These effects are likely the result of yeast overgrowth that occurs from ingesting sugary or high-glycemic types of foods. Furthermore, it is said that arthritis, allergies, asthma, psoriasis, eczema, fibromyalgia, cancer, and a host of other autoimmune disorders can be initiated and sustained by the consumption of sugar. Hormonal balance, also, can be disrupted in both men and women.

By removing sugar from your diet for the period of your Jump-Start Cleanse, you break the cycle of sugar addiction, resensitizing your glycogen receptors so that you get more energy from less food, eliminating the craving for sugar. You will also feel energized in a more consistent way, without the ups and downs inherent in sugar dependency.

When I say "avoid sugar," I also mean cut out honey, raw sugar, turbinado sugar, molasses, corn syrup, maple syrup, high fructose corn syrup, powdered sugar, malto-dextrin, mannitol, fructose, dextrose, glucose, maltose, sucrose (or any ingredient name ending in "-ose"), as well as artificial sweeteners. If you suffer frequent yeast or bacterial infections, you may want to consider giving up yeast at this time, as well. *Candida albicans* (a species of yeast) naturally occurs in the human body, but it can grow disproportionately, causing excess infections and other problems. It thrives on the consumption of sugars and yeast, so giving up yeast as you abstain from sugar will help alleviate candida-related issues (including gas, irritable bowel syndrome, heartburn, bad breath, headaches, congestion, dry or itchy skin, anxiety, fluid retention, and frequent urination).

In place of the aforementioned sweeteners, I recommend Stevia, a South American herb that the FDA has yet to approve as a sweetner and that is not commonly available in the UK. If you can find it, however, it has a negligible effect on blood sugar levels and even enhances glucose tolerance. Agave nectar is another delicious sweetner; it is low on the glycemic scale, so it's good for people with diabetes or insulin resistance or anyone watching his carbohydrate intake. Or you can try xylitol, a low-calorie natural sweetener extracted from birch bark and corn cobs, which is anti-microbial, and dissolves mucus, aiding in relief from inflammation. And similarly, it works well for those concerned with blood sugar and calories. Brown-rice syrup also works well to mildly sweeten things without causing a big spike in insulin. Just be sure to avoid all artificial sweeteners. Anytime you can choose something safe and natural over something processed and chemical, you are making the prudent choice.

Alcohol. Once consumed, alcohol is converted into glucose, or blood sugar, and causes many of the same physical problems as sugar consumption—in fact, alcohol and sugar are almost identical molecularly. Because they each have a similar high-and-low effect, it will be easier to abstain from consuming both at the same time than to try to eliminate just one. Beyond the sugar issues previously discussed, there are many reasons to take a break from alcohol consumption. Namely, alcohol depletes the brain of its natural mood-enhancing chemicals, can cause brain damage in large amounts, and can overload the liver with toxicity. Remarkably, nearly all these negative effects are remedied by taking a fast from alcohol.

The brain manufactures its own warehouse of mood-altering chemicals, including natural pain relievers, stimulants, and sedatives, which work in perfect harmony with the body and its chemistry. These naturally produced chemicals keep you feeling well-adjusted to your changing life and environment. Stress, especially extended periods of stress (the norm for many people), uses up these homemade chemicals rapidly. And considering that the volume of your own personal storehouse's production is determined by your genetic inheritance, it's possible that you didn't come into this world with the capacity to produce a whole lot of useful brain chemicals to begin with (you can look somewhat to your relatives' moods to determine this—cranky people? addicts? or happy and generally even-keeled?). If your brain's warehouse of chemicals can't keep up with your need for them, it will use its emergency storage. And once that's used up, you may find yourself turning to the druglike effects of alcohol (and some foods or prescription drugs) to help you feel okay.

This wouldn't be such a bad solution, except that when you drink alcohol, the important production centers in your brain get out of shape—just as a person would lose the ability to walk or lift heavy things if the body never did these things but had machines do them instead. The receptors that normally receive mood-altering chemicals produced by the brain, called neurotransmitters, instead receive the chemicals in the alcohol that you're consuming. Because these alcohol chemicals plug into your receptors the way your natural brain chemicals would, the production centers in your brain are sent the message that its receptors are full, and it should produce even less of its own chemicals.

You can see how this turns into a vicious circle. With a decline in the production of your own natural brain chemicals, your desire for quantities of alcohol will increase. Certainly everyone remembers how powerfully they felt the effect of their first drink, and as one matures, more and more alcohol is usually required to achieve that same effect. Because your brain's "in house"-produced chemicals are thousands of times stronger than anything you can find in the outside world, no matter how much you can drink, the alcohol loses its effectiveness. Unfortunately, by this time, your brain has slowed its production of its own chemicals significantly. So you may still crave a drink, but get less feeling from its consumption. Taking a break allows the receptors and producers in your brain to return to their natural call-and-response. Empty receptors send the message to production centers to produce greater volume. The need for neurotransmitters stimulates their production, and you'll begin to return to that natural-high place that you see in happy, healthy children.

As reported in the *Journal of Cell Biology*, researchers at Harvard Medical School have observed that the blood alcohol level achieved by just one drink is enough to inhibit cell-cell adhesion, causing permanent memory loss, weakening the brain's capacity to learn, and leading to various other memory disorders. Higher-order functions such as reasoning, planning, and prioritizing are also damaged, as a result of documented damage in the prefrontal cortex, the seat of higher reasoning. And that's just one drink.

Dr. Andreas Bartsch of the University of Würzberg in Germany conducted a groundbreaking study in which the human brain was studied for growth and regeneration as his subjects abstained from alcohol consumption. Bartsch and his team used magnetic resonance imaging (MRI) to assess and track key brain chemicals, and also gave their subjects tests of cognitive function. In consideration of this study's results, Bartsch stated, "Abstinence pays off and enables the brain to regain some substance and perform better. The adult human brain, and particularly its white matter, seems to possess genuine capabilities for regrowth."

And of course, alcohol is toxic to the body and especially hard on the liver. The free radicals in alcohol cause the liver to become inflamed, and this in itself leads to the production of scar tissue on the liver. Because the liver works like a sponge, hard and dense scar tissue coats and prevents the liver from functioning properly. When your liver doesn't function properly, the toxins it's trying to filter out of your bloodstream simply don't get filtered out. They can then wreak havoc on the rest of your body and your brain.

The liver does its best to break down alcohol into acetaldehyde, then into acetic acid, and then ideally into glucose, which enters the bloodstream, causing blood sugar levels to spike (see Sugar section). But both acetaldehyde and acetic acid are challenging for the liver to process, and it's not uncommon for the liver to be unable to deal with them right away. As a result, the liver will either release these chemicals back into the bloodstream, causing more toxic damage to the entire body than pure alcohol would, or it will valiantly and self-destructively hold on to the unprocessed acetic acid and/or acetalde-hyde by producing fatty tissues for storage. This leads to a less effective liver, and to liver damage.

Some signs of a weakened liver include body edema (swelling) and bruising. Another common sign is greater sensitivity to drugs and alcohol—you might be called a lightweight. Your liver may not be strong enough to filter out toxins from the bloodstream completely, and so they effect you more powerfully than they would someone with a healthy, fully functional liver.

Studies have looked at the possible health-giving benefits of both red and white wine. While the antioxidants present in these wines may benefit the heart and lungs respectively, the most profound ben-efit lies in the calming effect alcohol has on the entire nervous sys-tem. This calm affects the entire body in a healthful way, possibly prolonging life. This is a valid benefit, but know that this calm can be achieved through other means (like deep breathing and yoga)—at least during the period of your fast—and doesn't outweigh the benefits of abstaining from alcohol, briefly giving your body a rest from the other, less-beneficial effects. The National Institute on Alcohol Abuse and Alcoholism has reported several studies offering assurance that abstinence from alcohol is a highly effective means of allowing the liver to heal, regenerate, and cleanse itself.

By incorporating a break from alcohol into your Jump-Start Cleanse, you will be rebalancing your brain chemicals, healing brain damage, increasing your mental strength, and regenerating, toning, and purifying the liver.

Caffeine. The Royal College of Psychiatrists in the United Kingdom recently published an article suggesting that psychiatrists should routinely check for caffeine consumption when evaluating new patients. This is because consumption of caffeine leads to "symptoms which overlap with those of many psychiatric disorders," including, but not limited to, anxiety, sleep disorders, exacerbation of eating disorders, hostility, and other psychotic symptoms. The world's most popular psychoactive drug, according to Penn State's bio-behavioral health and pharmacology department, caffeine stimulates the central nervous system by tricking the brain into ordering the release of excess adrenaline. This excess adrenaline in your body builds up in your muscles, creating body tension, headaches, and muscle spasms. And because your adrenal glands are being artificially stimulated by a chemical (caffeine), they may not have ample time to rest and rejuvenate themselves, and may become depleted and weak. This, in turn, results in increased feelings of exhaustion, even when the brain is ordering the release of adrenaline (whether stimulated by caffeine or naturally). You may find you need more and more caffeine to feel awake or even normal.

Although caffeine is an addictive drug, you would have to consume (approximately) upwards of fifty cups of coffee in one day, obviously an unlikely amount, to die from this substance. However, even small quantities cause nervousness and can put you on a roller-coaster ride from a high to the inevitable low that follows. And giving up a heavy addiction to caffeine can involve withdrawal symptoms not unlike those experienced by cocaine addicts: headache, irritability, lethargy, nervousness, depression, and even drug-seeking behavior are not at all uncommon.

Giving up caffeine for the period of your cleanse will give your body a chance to replenish and restore your adrenal glands. Your adrenaline release will readjust itself, becoming more naturally in tune with your life and needs, as regulated by the brain rather than your coffee cup; your wise, innate physiology will naturally find the appropriate amount for each circumstance that arises in your day. Your body will be able to process the excess adrenaline stored in your muscles, leading to a greater sense of well-being, release of muscle tension and spasms, and fewer tension headaches. If you choose to return to your caffeine after your cleanse, you will need less of it, as your body will resensitize to it. You may find you have more energy than before, and no longer require a coffee or a soda to get yourself going.

Gluten. Gluten, a protein found in many foods, including wheat, barley, rye, and malt, is the most common irritant of the small intestine. Symptoms of irritation from gluten vary in degree from individual to individual, and gluten intolerance may be inherited. For most people, consumption of gluten can cause the immune system to attack the small intestine through inflammation, leading to gas, diarrhea, skin rashes, and may prevent the absorption of vital nutrients and vitamins, leading to depression and exhaustion. A gluten-heavy diet may contribute to osteoporosis, anemia, and vitamin and mineral deficiencies, primarily because the small intestine is too inflamed to perform its duty of absorbing nourishment.

Because gluten is so difficult to digest, it can leak, undigested, into the bloodstream. This phenomenon has become a topic in autism research, because undigested gluten has the ability to attach itself to the opiate receptors of the brain, mimicking the effect of a morphine high. In some of us, this manifests itself as the mild feeling of relaxation we associate with eating after consuming gluten-containing products like bread, pasta, or beer. But gluten can send some unlucky folks into an otherworldly opiate haze, as researchers in England, Norway, and the University of Florida have found in studies of those who suffer from autism. In fact, the Cure Autism Now! organization recommends that parents take autistic children off all gluten products for a period of at least three months, because of the remarkable success rate of those children who maintain a gluten-free diet. Children who made the dietary switch began making eye contact with their parents for the first time and attended non-special education classes in school. Research at the Johnson & Johnson Ortho-Clinical Diagnostics company has shown that casein, a protein found in milk, can have the same effect on the brain. These studies suggest that anything the body can interpret as an opiate can become addictive, and gluten is a major culprit, behaving like a powerful, mood-altering, brain-damaging drug.

Each individual has a different sensitivity to gluten, but almost everyone suffers some irritation from it. Abstaining from gluten for the period of your cleanse will allow the small intestine to soothe and heal itself, reestablishing its efficient absorption of nutrients. You will feel more energized, alert, and nourished.

Animal products. During the course of your fast you will also want to avoid all dairy, including milk, cheese, butter, sour cream, cream cheese, whipped cream, and any foods that contain these items. Dairy is full of lactose, a commonly indigestible allergen. Refraining from milk products during your fast will give your body a break from any inflammation you may be incurring from lactose.

Remember the quasi-opiate casein, discussed above? In the digestive tract, casein breaks down to produce peptides called casomorphines, which are opioids. In the brain, these compounds mimic opiate drugs like heroin or morphine, causing sleepiness and feelings of heaviness, but also stimulating a craving for more once the effect has worn off. Casein is also a histamine releaser, causing inflammation that can lead to premature aging and to diseases like cancer.

Casein is a major topic in *The China Study*, in which Dr. T. Colin Campbell describes how casein promotes cancer in all the disease's stages of development. If you consider the original purpose of cow's milk, to feed calves, who have four stomachs and will double their weight in forty-seven days, it's clear that the growth-promoting properties of milk are not appropriate for other animals, especially humans. In fact, these very growth-promoting properties end up being used as stimulation not only for growth of the body but also for the proliferation and growth of cancer cells.

Campbell's studies garnered so much attention, that a collaboration between Cornell and Oxford Universities and China's national health research laboratory was undertaken to study the effect of casein and other animal proteins on a broad base of human subjects. The results were astounding, with consumption of animal proteins directly linked to the development of cancer and several other diseases.

Casein is not only present in milk, but is also the main ingredient in many soy cheeses. It's a powerful binder, and not easily destroyed (or digested), so it's also a common food additive in processed snacks. It's found in soups, protein powders, cereal, infant formula, energy bars, salad dressings, and even some vegetarian meats. You may be disturbed to know that this same so-called edible ingredient, which is commonly known to be difficult to digest, is also a primary ingredient in glues, protective coatings, plastics, and fabrics. The University of Berlin recently showed, in a study published in the *European Heart Journal*, that simply adding milk to tea blocks any health benefits the tea might have (particularly cardiovascular), because the casein binds to the other molecules in the tea, rendering them useless. Casein acts like a glue no matter where it goes, including the human body. It stimulates the production of mucus and binds to the mucus, making it thicker and more troublesome.

Dairy is also polluted by the industrial processing of cows, including antibiotics, hormones, and unnatural feed. As any breastfeeding mother can tell you, what the mother eats will show up in the milk she produces. If a woman who is nursing drinks coffee before she feeds her child, you can bet her baby will be wide awake for hours. Similarly, what is fed to cows goes into their milk, and this includes synthetic and naturally occurring hormones and antibiotics. Humans who consume dairy products are consuming these as well. Even organic milk contains hormones, though usually not the artificial bovine growth hormone.

The industrial processing of animals has corrupted not only dairy products but meats as well. While some meats have beneficial nutrients, such as the omega-3 fatty acids in salmon or the iron in egg yolks, the industrial age has created an environment where the potential damage to your health from meats outweighs any benefit they may have. Oceans, rivers, and lakes are polluted beyond our ability to measure; when you eat animals from the water, there's no way to know what you're getting. The Food and Drug Administration (FDA) and the Environmental Protection Agency (EPA) have advised pregnant women, nursing mothers, and young children to abstain from eating shark, swordfish, king mackerel, and tilefish, due to their high levels of highly toxic and damaging mercury, among other heavy metals. Shellfish (such as shrimp), canned light tuna, salmon, pollock, and catfish should to be limited to twelve ounces per week because of their heavy-metal content. The effects of mercury are partially reversible in adults, but permanent damage will be sustained by children who are still developing. Both the EPA and the FDA admit that they just can't determine how much mercury or other heavy metals are in these fish, as amounts vary from fish to fish, and the industry is not adequately regulated.

When you purchase fish at the market or are served in a restaurant, you can't always be sure where that fish was caught or how it was processed. Human and industrial pollution to our water is so out of control, we simply do not know what kind of industrial waste any particular fish has absorbed or ingested. Coal-burning power plants release mercury in their smoke, and that mercury pours into our waters when it rains. Heavy metals are the most dangerous pollutants we consume. They are not water soluble, and so are indigestible. They may remain in the body indefinitely, leading to nerve damage, neurological issues such as numbness in the arms and legs, learning disabilities, kidney damage, and hearing and vision loss. The best way to prevent mercury buildup in your system is to stop consuming it and allow the body to purify itself.

Unlike fish, farm-raised meats might seem more controllable, and perhaps more likely to remain pure. On the contrary: most farm-raised meats exist in such tight quarters that the animals' natural eliminative processes are hindered. They have no exercise, so the growth hormones, antibiotics, and other chemicals with which they're injected or fed are not fully processed out of their bodies. It all stays in the meat. That puts the burden on *your* body to eliminate these toxins, and that's no easy task.

Much of the meat and dairy we consume is nutritionally compromised or even harmful at the point of purchase. To make matters worse, various studies point to the toxic effects of cooking animal products. The University of Toronto and the *Journal of the National Cancer Institute* have each published articles relating the ingestion of cooked and pasteurized dairy products to an increased risk of colon cancer. The proteins found naturally in meats are somewhat fragile substances, and when exposed to heat, the protein molecules reorganize themselves in a way that is not only difficult to digest and enzyme-depleting, but toxic to the human body. Several studies done since the heating of muscle meat was first discovered to be cancer causing, in 1990, have proved again and again that heterocyclic amines (HCAs), also carcinogenic, are created when muscle meat is cooked.

While cooked animal products are clearly not beneficial, I can't recommend incorporating raw animal products in your cleanse, either. Without the benefit of heat, meat, fish, and dairy products are dangerous because of the bacteria and parasites they contain. So at least while you're purifying, for your own safety, cut out animal products altogether.

By going dairy-free for the period of your fast, you're avoiding a major allergen (lactose) and allowing your body to get rid of its irritation. Also, you're giving the body a chance to process and eliminate any casein gumming up your system. You are most likely preventing cancer, and giving your body a chance to process out the toxic chemicals present in milk and its by-products. By eliminating meats and seafood, you're giving your body a break from the onslaught of industrial pollutants, antibiotics, hormones, and chemicals inherent in modern-day livestock and fish production. This reprieve will also enable your body to recover from free-radical damage associated with ingestion of meat-related carcinogens.

At this point you may be asking, what *can* I have?

Water. The most important thing to put into your body during your cleanse is pure water. And not just during a cleanse. We tend not to drink nearly enough water, even though bottled water sales have soared in recent years. Water helps remove waste from cells and aids fat metabolism; it keeps our brains functioning properly and lubricates and flushes our systems. Water is important for transporting nutrients and wastes, regulating our body temperature, and helping our tissues stay healthy and strong.

During your cleanse, try to drink at least two quarts of plain water a day to assist your kidneys in cleaning the toxins out of your blood.

Fresh, whole foods. Eating lots of fresh, raw salads is like sending scrubbing brushes through your digestive system, clearing away old, undigested foods, dead tissues, and mucus. Try integrating brown rice and quinoa, steamed or sautéed vegetables, miso soup with rice noodles, buckwheat pancakes made with rice milk, and lots of fresh fruits and fruit smoothies. I also enjoy rice cakes with nut butter spread on them, hearty soups made with beans and vegetables, hot cereals with nuts and chopped up apples or pears on top, grilled or stir-fried vegetables and sweet potatoes served with tofu and a nice marinade (there are many delicious and wholesome premade ones available at health food stores). I love avocados, and since they have a lot of protein and good fat in them, I slice them up and spread them over a piece of whole grain toast or flax cracker and put tomatoes and sprouts on top for a nice sandwich. Once you open your mind to new foods, the choices are endless.

Get a massage, soak in a tub. To further support your efforts during the period of your fast, enjoy the healing and cleansing benefits of massage, yoga, and hot baths in mineral salts (Dead Sea salts are known to have the highest mineral content). These three practices have a powerful effect on the body, drawing toxins out of the deepest places—organs, muscles, and fat—and assisting in their removal from the body. Colonic therapy is also deeply cleansing, removing undigested substances from the colon, decreasing the likelihood of colon cancer and numerous other maladies. Benefits of colon cleansing include fresher breath, less body odor, a flatter belly, better regularity, and weight loss.

Also, try to avoid any toxic substances you have around the house and in your personal-care products. You can check the Suggested Reading and Viewing section at the end of this book for websites that will list particularly toxic chemicals to avoid.

Try this:

Eliminate sugar, alcohol, caffeine, gluten, and animal products from your diet for anywhere from a week to twenty-one days. Eat only fresh, whole foods and drink lots of water, and take a hot bath or get a massage. By adhering to this cleanse you will clear your body of some potential allergens, toxins, addictions, and carcinogens. This brief practice alone will reset your body's functions and point you directly toward greater health, vitality, and energy.

CHAPTER SIX

Your Nest
Creating a Magical Environment

IT'S VERY NATURAL, AS YOU BEGIN TO TUNE IN TO YOUR BODY AND YOUR emotions and start being more aware of what is and isn't working in your life, to feel an urge to get rid of things that are no longer useful. Your physical environment is an extension of your body and mind, and it will reflect what's going on with you—and vice versa. Being in a space that feels good will go a long way in creating a positive experience of wellness.

When you're in a rut, you tend to see the world through a lens of "things are not quite right and I feel ill at ease," whereas when you look around and feel comfortable and inspired, you tend to see the world through eyes that tell you "all is well and I'm feeling particularly creative and enthusiastic about life." It's really important that your surroundings reflect and inspire that latter aspect of your soul.

Of course, much of this perception is subtle; we respond to light, space, and pleasing visuals without necessarily zeroing in on what it is that sets the tone. But our environment does indeed set the tone and serve as a backdrop for our life. You can walk through a door and feel soured by the energy that is all around, or you can walk into a place that seems to sing to your soul. Once you learn how you respond to different parts of your physical environment, you can make adjustments accordingly and experience an almost immediate upgrade in your well-being. As always, it starts with paying attention, and it's pretty simple after that.

Take a look around at your physical space and ask yourself a few questions:

Do you feel nurtured or drained by being there? Is it cozy and welcoming? Cluttered? Cold or warm? Light or dark?

Remember, there are no right or wrong answers to these questions; you just want to be aware of the many ways that your space affects your sense of well-being.

I once lived in a large apartment in New York City that I had lusted after for many years before I was finally able to move in. The place had all the goodies—a doorman, roof garden, and a washer and dryer right in the apartment (a big deal in New York City), and it was located in a very chic part of town. The place was amazing, which was why it baffled me to no end that I always found myself getting depressed there. I finally realized that as beautiful and tony as the apartment was, it was also quite dark. I am someone who thrives in a bright space, and so no matter how impressive the address was, it just didn't work for me.

I came to the conclusion that I would much rather be in a small apartment with lots of light than a big place that was on the darker side. I also realized that city living made me a little anxious, and so I began to move my life more toward spending time in the country, with the eventual goal of living someplace quiet and rural.

These were, of course, big decisions to make, and I realize what a privilege it was for me to have so many choices. You may recognize that your space isn't working for you but be unable to pick up and move. But there are many ways to make adjustments. Some good lamps might have helped my New York apartment! The point is, I wasn't even aware of my need for light until I found myself depressed in that dark place.

Awareness is the precursor to change. So keep checking in with yourself to see if you are living in a way that authentically feeds your soul and sense of well-being. To thrive as we move along our continuum of wellness and enlightenment, we must feel embraced by the physical space we spend so much time in.

Exercise: When Was the Last Time I Even Looked at This?

In the spirit of clearing away the old to make room for the new, take a look around your home and notice what you like and don't like about the space you live in. What brings you the most joy, and what doesn't seem right? Maybe a particular object or choice never pleased you, or maybe you've just grown tired of it or it no longer reflects who you are. My friend Robin has a beautiful little cottage in a suburb outside the city. When Robin's mother died, she left Robin all the contents of her home, and since Robin was an up-and-coming artist, she joyfully placed the furniture throughout the house until it was all filled up and looked lived in. Finally she had dishes and glassware for entertaining; she had a real desk with antique chairs that made the place appear sturdy and settled; and she had exotic, well-collected-looking knickknacks from her mother's travels.

After a few months of enjoying her new "adult" home, Robin realized she had not gotten much done in the way of painting. Every time she went to the easel, she started thinking of other things that took away her creative mojo. Soon Robin noticed that the energy around her had shifted. Her home was no longer hers; it felt like leftover energy from her mother's life. Even though she loved her mother very much and had no bad memories or feelings about her, she just didn't feel that the place nurtured her own developing creative spirit. So, as much as it seemed wasteful at first, Robin went about giving away (to people who very much appreciated them) most of the items that she had installed in the cottage. She kept a few key things—the cookware that her mother had used to make Robin lunches and dinners over the years, some picture frames that held the family history, and a tiny chair that Robin had used as a child—and she cleared the rest out in the spirit of making her home her own.

Sure enough, Robin began to paint again. Her home was a lot sparer now but had that wide-open feeling that worked well for an artist. Robin felt like she was "in her own skin," and she thrived.

Even if something has undisputed value on paper, you might consider letting it go if it doesn't add to your feeling of comfort, safety, joy, and inspiration.

Sometimes I have clients go through a little exercise in which they look at their possessions and ask themselves, *When was the last time I touched this? Do I still need it in my life?* If you haven't touched or used or gotten pleasure out of looking at something in a year or more, it's probable that you could let it go without mourning its absence. If you don't use it, maybe someone else could. Give it away!

When I made the shift to being vegan, I went through my closets and got rid of everything that had fur trim on it (quite a few things, I'm ashamed to admit) or was made from an exotic animal skin like alligator or ostrich. I had experienced this enormous shift in consciousness when I gave up eating meat, and it felt good to clear out the reminders of my old ways.

I will admit that it was a little harder to get rid of my favorite shoes (I gave up buying leather after seeing how greatly cows suffered for our little luxuries), but I did so in waves. I kept aside the shoes that I wore regularly, and then gradually, over the years, cleared them out and replaced them with nonleather ones (which I have to say are just as fabulous!).

In clearing your space, you are acknowledging that you are moving forward out of an old stage and into a new phase. This honing of your possessions represents a significant inner shift toward being streamlined and light. Let things go joyfully, knowing that a higher vibration is soon to take their place.

Let Go of High-Maintenance Possessions

Another helpful thing to do to free up your energy is identify your high-maintenance possessions and determine if they are worth all the time and energy you have to put into them. For me, it was my complicated stereo system. I always had a hard time with it. It seemed to have a mind of its own and went on the fritz (or maybe I fritzed it!) a couple of times a year, which required that I track down a shop that could fix it, then schlep it in, leaving it for a couple of weeks while hoping that the bill wouldn't get too high. More often than not, I needed some new part or component that would make it all work better.

Once I identified that the stereo was taking more from me than it was giving back, I decided to give it away. These days I rely on my little iPod and speakers, which give me just as much listening pleasure without all the hassle and stress. Some things, of course, require a lot of maintenance but bring us great joy—say an antique car or a lovely garden. If that's the case, they're obviously worth keeping.

Weed Out What's Outdated or Stale

As you work on clearing your home or office, weed out the obvious things, such as books you don't like or wouldn't care to read or refer to again. Get rid of old magazines and papers that are lying around. Clear out your toiletry cabinets and ditch expired medications. Go through the refrigerator and pantry and pitch anything that is unhealthy or that's been sitting too long. Look at the labels on your various cleansers and cleaning agents and toss out the ones that are full of chemicals with unpronounceable names. Open your closets and garage and be vigilant in going through everything. It's amazing how much you can throw away once you get started.

And most importantly, tie up all the loose ends you come across. File away what's sitting on your desk; follow up on projects you have in your to-do box; and return the outstanding e-mails or phone calls that nag at you.

If you find yourself resisting following through on something, you might want to consider putting closure on whatever it is, whether it's a friend you are hesitant to stay in touch with or a potential job situation that just doesn't feel right. Sometimes it is enormously freeing just to say, "This is no longer part of my path; I choose to let it go." Once you tend to it lovingly and with firm detachment, get all the reminders of it out of your space so that it no longer tugs at your attention and makes you feel guilty.

Now Comes the Fun Part: Re-create Your Space

After clearing away the clutter and extraneous things, you may begin to see greater potential for your living space. This is the time to ask yourself what you want to express with your space.

Personally, I want to feel peaceful and in touch with Spirit and nature, so my home reflects all that. I like to be reminded of my spiritual interests every day, so I enjoy candles, paintings that have a mystical message within them, and freshly cut flowers.

Some people prefer more architectural lines to reflect their vision of order and design, while others might want to be surrounded by books so that they are reminded of all the things they have learned.

Transforming your living space from a place that is simply functional into something that is more sacred and nourishing is a powerful step in upgrading your energy. Even if you have kids, chaos, and a house that is not quite your ideal, you can still elicit a significant shift by keeping the following in mind:

- **Throw out old stuff.**

- **Cease buying things just for the sake of buying something new.**

- **Only add items that make you feel joy when you are around them (or things that you truly need, like cleaning supplies).**

- **Switch over to natural products to clean and keep up your home. The fewer chemicals there are in the solutions the better.**

- **The same goes for toiletries and makeup. There are so many new options available online and in natural foods stores; it's just a matter of trying different brands until you find the ones you like.**

- **As much as you can, keep it simple.**

Adding a Home Altar

I enjoy having an altar in my house. For me, it always pulls my energy back to what is important and meaningful. It can be just a small stand (or table) decorated with relics that represent all the important aspects of a fulfilling life. I have things that represent spirituality (a statue of Jesus, a figurine of the Buddha, a rosary, and some prayer beads that a monk gave me in Burma), health (seasonal flowers, which signify fresh air and sunshine), abundance (some pretty shells from my favorite beach trip and a few coins I picked up on the street when I was feeling lucky), romance (my favorite love poem and a red candle), and dharma, or life's purposeful work (a picture of some children my husband and I put through school).

Every time I pass by my altar, I am reminded of what is important and to bring my focus back to my core values. I make a practice of meditating in front of it once a day for about twenty minutes, and while I'm home, I keep the candle (and sometimes incense) burning so that the energy of it feels active; it helps me to feel in touch with my higher purpose, personal motivations, and sources of empowerment.

Try this:

1. **Look at your home environment with fresh eyes. Think about what you want your home space to reflect about you, and whether it does that.**

2. **Get rid of old things that you don't use or love anymore; let go of high-maintenance items that drain you.**

3. **Only bring in new things that nourish your sense of wellness and fulfillment. This includes cleaning products, toiletries, and cosmetics.**

4. **Construct an altar in your space to help you stay in touch with important elements of who you truly are and where you're going: spiritual reverence, personal inspirations, purpose, heart, gratitude, motivation, and sources of empowerment.**

PART THREE

Laying the Groundwork

CHAPTER SEVEN

Give Us This Day . . .
Considering the Health, Environmental, and Spiritual Implications of the Foods We Choose to Eat

IN THE PAST FEW CHAPTERS WE'VE BEEN WORKING ON CLEARING AND cleaning. You've done a body cleanse and looked at your living and working environments with fresh eyes. From the various cleanses and clearings, you are, I hope, feeling lighter physically and emotionally, and are more aware of what brings you to higher levels of wellness and what drags you back down. One of those drags is bad fuel. In this next section we'll look at the positive practices that support our health and vitality in the long term and that, over time, will bump us up to higher and higher levels of wellness.

Just as you wouldn't expect your car to run on bad fuel, you can't expect to feel extraordinary if you're not eating well. I like to call this pillar of wellness cross-training "conscious eating." When we eat consciously—considering the entire picture—we need to look at every aspect of the foods we eat: how they serve our bodies, where they come from, and how they got to our plates.

As always, this is not about perfection but about leaning in the direction of change and making better and better choices. Quantum wellness, when it comes to eating, is about keeping your eyes open and scrutinizing the process from beginning to end, as well as thinking about how your dietary choices affect others. You want to eat in a way that is not only good for you but good for everyone involved in bringing your food to you: workers on all levels of production, the animals, and the environment as a whole.

Any food choice that is truly good for your health will also be beneficial to your spiritual well-being (meaning that no spiritual principles, such as mercy, compassion, environmental stewardship, or kindness, have been violated). When I think about eating consciously to support our bodies, our minds, our spirits, and the world around us, I often think of Marianne Williamson, the spiritual teacher and author, who says, "If God is smart enough to have created the universe, and keep the planets revolving around the sun, He can certainly handle the details of your little life." I would apply that wisdom here as well. If Spirit created us to need protein or iron or whatnot, that Source certainly would have provided a way for us to get it without causing pain or suffering to others.

Eating the "omnivorous" diet that is a part of our modern culture requires that we wear blinders to the immense suffering involved in delivering animal protein to our plates. Can you imagine Spirit (indulge me while I personalize this energy for a moment) saying, "Here, eat this bird because it has lots of protein and protein is essential for your health. Unfortunately, the people who raised that animal were treated just a few degrees better than serfs in feudal England, and the people who slaughtered her were treated in ways that, according to Human Rights Watch, violated their basic human rights. Also, the manure from that chicken, awash in bacteria, pesticides, herbicides, and antibiotics, well, it seems destined for the Chesapeake Bay, where it will create a new level 4 biohazard called Pfiesteria (a.k.a. "the cell from hell"). Oh, and finally, that chicken, who was once a cute little baby chick, led a miserable life from day one and suffered horrendous conditions until the day she was killed. I wish there was some other way for you to get your protein, but there isn't. So go ahead. Eat the chicken; grill it up and put some sauce on it and forget about all the other stuff and enjoy it because, hey, you need your protein."

No. If there is Spirit involved in the creation of the universe, certainly there exists a way to have food that enables us to be well fed, healthy, *and* kind to humans, the environment, and animals—all at the same time. This would be an all-around wise food choice, a quantum step for all.

Our task as thoughtful and evolving human beings is to determine our health in an integrated way. We can heed what the body needs *and* live in alignment with our spiritual interests. We live in a time when it's easier to access more choices, but it takes breaking out of old habits and traditions. We can examine our consumer behavior and then change it for the betterment of all concerned. It may require more attention and effort to be mindful of our food choices, but that's part of the fun (remember, fun is one of our cross-training tools!) and the power of living consciously—making every meal a "moment of being."

It's true that restaurants and grocery stores are only beginning to accommodate the requests of those who want a more interesting plant-based diet, but those who do make the requests lead the way. They see a future of peace and wellness on a global scale and are willing to be the pioneers in cultivating a practical philosophy of leading an examined and mindful life that reveres all living things.

Our evolution in human morality is marked almost entirely by our attempt to move beyond doing something simply because that's how we've always done it. Speaking in more explicitly ethical terms, we would be wise to fully reject the "might makes right" law of the jungle. It may indeed be "natural" for the powerful to dominate the weak (e.g. through slavery, murder, and subjugation of women and children), but that doesn't mean we should give in to that baser instinct.

If a food choice is really good for your health, it will also support your emotional and spiritual wellness. And vice versa. No one should have to cringe when they peer into the reality of where their food came from; we should instead feel inspired knowing that we are waking up to a deeper and more responsible connectedness with all life. As Albert Einstein wisely said, "Our task must be to free ourselves . . . by widening our circle of compassion to embrace all living creatures and the whole of nature and its beauty." Or as Saint Paul wrote to the Galatians* (NRSV), "You reap whatever you sow." By orienting ourselves toward conscious eating we will not only push forward our spiritual growth and physical wellness, but we will also do an enormous service in bringing about a kinder and more peaceful world.

There's a lot to think about, and I'm sure you are tired of seeing fear-inducing articles in the paper every week about which foods are safe and which ones aren't. It's hard to navigate the abundance of nutritional advice and feel like you know what you're doing. But one basic principle that remains constant is this: the closer your food is to its source—and the closer you are to being aware of the process of getting it to you—the better it will be for you. Whole foods harvested thoughtfully are *always*—yes, always—the better choice.

The food we eat today comes to us in a radically different manner than it did even fifty years ago. Our food is not only grown with more hormones, antibiotics, and chemicals than ever before, but it is also more processed, more packaged, and transported greater distances than ever before. Small family-run farms are going extinct, giving way to corporate factory farms that are driven, it seems, almost solely by the desire for profit. Values of stewardship of the land and

---

*Unless otherwise noted, all biblical quotations are taken from the New Revised Standard Version.

all its inhabitants, accountability to one's community, and pride in producing something that tastes wonderful—all these basic values seem to have become the exception rather than the rule. Yes, we are seeing a swing back to these values, and may the trend blossom into a consumer force to be reckoned with.

Because everything is indeed connected, what behooves us spiritually also improves our health and the world around us. Eastern spirituality teaches about the love infused in our food. The belief behind this is that food is more than core nutrients; it is also the work that went into it. When food is produced in a fair and just way by people who take pride in their work, the food is better. The reverse, of course, is also true: if there are blood, sweat, and tears (as well as a heavy dose of cruelty to animals and environmental havoc) involved in producing food, that negativity will flow directly into the food as well.

It can be deeply disturbing to investigate the ramifications of how our provisions came to our plate, but if we want to experience wellness and evolve to a higher state of being human, we are obliged to do this work. That is part of the Socratic idea of leading an examined life.

Vegetarianism: The Ethical Issues

For many years I had two books on my to-read list that I was too scared to touch: *Animal Factories*, coauthored by investigative journalist Jim Mason and the controversial Princeton philosopher Peter Singer, whom the *New York Times* has called the most influential living philosopher; and *Diet for a New America*, by Baskin-Robbins heir John Robbins, about the effect of raising animals for food on our health, the environment, and the animals themselves.

It's not that I was even an animal lover, per se. I liked my dogs and took good care of them, but it was so much easier not to think about the suffering of other animals (farm animals). Even so, I did know that these creatures were not inanimate objects; they had individual traits and characteristics that made me think that they had been given life by the same Creator that gave me life. All the major wisdom philosophies teach kindness and compassion, and it is a basic tenet of all religions that we humans should extend love and refrain from causing pain. Would it not then be imperative to consider that by continuing to eat meat we are causing great suffering and pain? And needlessly at that? Regardless of your religious or spiritual leanings, this mandate not to cause pain seems a matter of basic human decency.

As hard as we may try to avoid thinking about it, the fact is, animals are made of the same basic elements as humans—if you prick them, they bleed. They are real living, sentient beings. Whether mammal, bird, or fish, we all touch, taste, see, hear, and smell in varying degrees. Look into a goat's eyes or see the tenderness between a mother cow and her calf and you will find something sacred and lovely.

Perhaps you are like me. For a very long time I didn't want to know the details of what went into making my favorite meals. But as I grew in my spiritual life, I realized that I could no longer ignore my own hypocrisy on this subject. If I was going to continue to eat meat, the least I could do was know what it was I was supporting with that choice. So with a deep breath, I picked up *Animal Factories* and read it. Then I read *Diet for a New America*. And then I read *Animal Theology*, by the Oxford University theology professor and Anglican priest Dr. Andrew Linzey, who looks at animal rights from a Christian viewpoint. And then I moved on to *Slaughterhouse: The Shocking Story of Greed, Neglect, and Inhumane Treatment Inside the U.S. Meat Industry,* by Gail Eisnitz. A few quotations from factory-farm workers put me over the edge:

"One time the knocking gun was broke all day, they were taking a knife and cutting the back of the cow's neck open while he's still standing up. They would just fall down and be shaking. And they stab cows in the butt to make 'em move. Break their tails. Beat them so bad. I've drug cows til their bones start breaking, while they're still alive. Bringing them around the corner and they get stuck up in the doorway, just pull them till their hide be ripped, til the blood just drip on the steel and concrete. Breaking their legs pulling them in. And the cow be crying with its tongue stuck out. They pull him till his neck just pops."

"To keep that production line moving . . . quite often uncooperative animals are beaten, they have prods poked in their faces, and up their rectums, they have bones broken and eyeballs popped out."

"Dragging cattle with a chain and forklift is a standard practice at the plant," explained a long-term inspector at a large beef operation in Nebraska, "and that's even after the forklift operator rolled over and crushed the head of one downer while dragging another.". . . "[T]hey'll go through the skinning process alive. I saw that myself, a bunch of times. I've found them alive clear over to the rump stand. . . . And that happens in every plant. I've worked in four large ones and a bunch of small ones. They're all the same. . . . [E]verybody gets so used to it that it doesn't mean anything."

"In the summertime when it's ninety, ninety-five degrees, they're transporting cattle from twelve to fifteen hundred miles away on a trailer forty to forty-five head crammed in there, and some collapse from heat exhaustion. This past winter we had minus fifty degree weather with the windchill. Can you imagine if you were in the back of a trailer that's open and the windchill is minus fifty degrees, and that trailer is going fifty miles an hour? The animals are urinating and defecating right in the trailers, and after a while it's going to freeze, and their hooves are right in it. If they go down—well, you can imagine lying in there for ten hours on a trip."

"[O]ur legger gets beef that's still conscious all the time. Sometimes almost every one . . . I've seen beef still alive at the flankers, more often at the 'ears and horns.' That's a long way." . . . "They drag the live ones who can't stand up anymore out of the crate. They put a metal snare around her ear or foot and drag her the full length of the building. These animals are just screaming in pain." . . . "Worn out sows are then dumped on a pile, where they stay—for up to two weeks—until the cull truck picks them up."

All this so I could have my steak or chicken dinner?

Now unwilling to turn my back and motivated to learn all I could, I sat down and watched two films: *To Love or Kill: Man vs. Animal* directed by Anthony Thomas and *The Animals Film,* directed by Myriam Alaux and Victor Schonfeld, both of which explore how animals are used and misused for food, clothing, entertainment, and experimentation. And I kept going, agonizing as I read and studied and watched everything I could find on the subject of our treatment of animals for food and other consumer goods (fur, cosmetics, etc.).

When I had had more than I could take, I fell into a deep depression and wondered what I was supposed to do. Become vegetarian? Vegan? Join an animal activist group? I was shocked and overwhelmed and wondered what difference one person could even make. Anything I did seemed like it would just be a drop in the bucket. We are a meat-eating society and not about to shift direction overnight. Moreover, animal agriculture is big business—more than $100 billion a year, with the most powerful lobbying interest in Washington, even more powerful than the oil and pharmaceutical lobbies, as it was admirably exposed by investigative journalist and author Eric Schlosser, first in his book *Fast Food Nation,* and more recently in the *New York Times* and *Vanity Fair.* Not for nothing are we shown commercials and pictures of happy cows and clucky chickens frolicking in fields or nestling into cozy straw beds in bright red barns.

How many times did I shop for chicken breasts or baby back ribs without thinking about what those words really meant? I'm ashamed to say that it never really occurred to me until I saw some of those undercover videos. Ribs from a baby's back? A leg of a lamb? I finally had to just pause and allow the reality to gel in my mind.

It is a rude awakening, realizing that our diet is based in cruelty. Even buying humanely raised products is complicated, but current-day practices in industrial agriculture, especially in the raising and slaughter of animals for food, is a tragedy on an almost unimaginably huge scale. According to the United States Department of Agriculture (USDA), about 10 billion land animals (35 million cattle, 100 million pigs, 300 million turkeys, and about 9.5 billion chickens) are killed each year for food. Estimates of the number of fish killed are hard to come by, but one estimate of the number of fin fish killed every year for U.S. consumers alone is about 5 billion (plus 10 billion shellfish).

Try to imagine, for a moment, the ingenuity and speed that is required to process that many creatures "efficiently" and cost-effectively. Pig slaughter lines kill more than 1,000 animals per hour, and chicken slaughter lines kill even more. You can hardly blame workers in these factory settings for having thick skins and closed hearts. How else could they do it? But undercover investigations have shown that with this shutting down of consciousness on the part of the workers in these plants has come a blind eye toward and even a penchant for inflicting horrible abuses on the captive animals—from ripping the animals limb from limb, to blowing them up with dry-ice bombs, to raping them with metal gate rods, to skinning them alive and dropping cinder blocks on their heads.

These practices are not exceptional or isolated incidents; every time investigators go undercover, they find the most horrific abuses, and the consistent discoveries of sadistic cruelty in modern farms and slaughterhouses has become so overwhelming that the industry's claims of a few errant workers are becoming harder and harder to believe.

But even the standard abuses that the industry can't and doesn't deny will horrify any person who opposes cruelty to animals—and we all do, of course. The universal practices in modern farms and slaughterhouses would warrant felony charges if dogs or cats were their targets. Routinely, factory-farmed animals have their beaks, testicles, or horns chopped off without pain relief. They're crammed into cages and crates and massive warehouses in their own filth and are never allowed to do anything they wish to do. Mother pigs and almost all egg-laying hens cannot turn around or lie down comfortably. One can imagine them going out of their minds from the frustration and discomfort combined with the noises and smells and sights going on all around them.

This dreadfulness goes on at every moment of every day year after year after year. Once you allow yourself the awareness, it's hard to get it out of your mind (at least it was for me—impossible, actually), which is no doubt why so many of us avoid the topic. But if we want to be a part of the push toward a new level of conscious evolution, we simply can't hide our heads in the sand.

Vegetarianism: The Health Issues

As you know, the central theme of this book is that if something is good in one area of your life, it will be good in other areas. Eating a plant-based diet certainly adheres to this theme, since a plant-based diet is also extremely healthy.

Shockingly, more than half of all Americans die of heart disease or cancer, and two-thirds of us are overweight. The vast majority of the obesity and a lot of the heart disease and cancer is preventable through simple lifestyle and dietary choices. Indeed, the American Dietetic Association says that vegetarians have "lower rates of death from ischemic heart disease, . . . lower blood cholesterol levels, lower blood pressure, and lower rates of hypertension, type 2 diabetes, and prostate and colon cancer." Vegetarians, on average, are about one-third as likely to be overweight as meat eaters, and pure vegetarians (vegans) are about one-tenth as likely to be obese.

The reasons vegetarians have a major health advantage are simple: a sensible, natural, plant-based diet is packed with vitamins, minerals, antioxidants, healthy plant protein, fiber, and complex carbohydrates. Meat, including fish and chicken, is totally devoid of fiber and complex carbohydrates, and contains artery-clogging cholesterol, saturated animal fats, and toxic animal protein (more on this below), contaminated at alarmingly high rates with antibiotics, concentrated pesticide residues, hormones, and dangerous contaminants such as E. coli, salmonella, and campylobacter. (The vast majority of food poisoning cases in the U.S. are traceable to animal products.)

As I learned from Dr. Andrew Weil, among the many problems with meat is something called arachidonic acid, or AA. AA is a pro-inflammatory fatty acid that is found only in animal products. Dr. Weil explains that "heart disease and Alzheimer's—among many other diseases—begin as inflammatory processes. The same hormonal imbalance that increases inflammation also increases cell proliferation and the risk of malignant transformation." We are discovering that inflammation is really key in so many of the diseases that plague us. So when you eat meat, and Dr. Weil points out that even chicken is full of arachidonic acid, you are stoking the fires of the disease process. It doesn't matter if the chicken is free-range or the beef is grass-fed. The offending fatty acid is natural and inherent in the meat.

Arachidonic acid is a protein, so Dr. Weil's findings jibe with the thesis of one of my favorite books, *The China Study*, mentioned in chapter five. Please, if you have not read it yet, order it right now, and read it as soon as you're done with this book. There is no sadness in it, no horror stories or guilt trips—only an extremely thorough study of how animal protein affects your health and longevity. In a nutshell, the country's top nutritional researcher, Dr. T. Colin Campbell, a professor emeritus of nutritional biochemistry at Cornell University, pores over all the evidence presented to date (his is the most comprehensive survey of the connection between diet and disease in medical history), and argues with overwhelming evidence that "the data from the China Study suggest that what we have come to consider as 'normal' illnesses of aging are really not normal. In fact, these findings indicate that the vast majority, perhaps 80 to 90 percent of all cancers, cardiovascular diseases, and other forms of degenerative illness can be prevented, at least until very old age, simply by adopting a plant-based diet."

These are strong words from a man who grew up on a dairy farm, got his Ph.D. in animal nutrition, and worked on a project to produce animal protein more efficiently. According to Campbell, in addition to causing cancer, animal protein also fuels cancer that already exists. So you can have a carcinogen in your body, but it doesn't get "turned on" until you ingest animal flesh. Animal protein causes the carcinogen to become active and wreak havoc in the body. Even so-called lean cuts of meat such as fish and chicken are high in fat and protein, and as Campbell says, animal protein only causes "mischief."

Okay, I know the old joke: vegetarians don't live longer; it just *seems* longer to them, because they're living lives of deprivation. Well, it turns out that vegetarian lives are both longer and better. As for having strength and energy on a vegetarian diet, everyone I know who has adopted the diet testifies to having more energy, needing less sleep, feeling younger, and just having a more vibrant demeanor. In fact, some of the world's top athletes are vegetarian. Vegetarian athletes have the advantage of getting all the plant protein, complex carbohydrates, and fiber they need without all the artery-clogging saturated animal fats found in meat that would slow them down.

All that and it's a kinder way to live, too.

Vegetarianism: The Environmental Issues

There are great environmental costs to a meat-based diet as well. Thirty years ago, Frances Moore Lappé published her groundbreaking *Diet for a Small Planet*, which looks at the environmental consequences of funneling crops through animals, as well as the consequences of first-world meat consumption on global poverty and destitution. Lappé's statistics hold up today as well. Eating meat is incredibly inefficient and wasteful. It takes many pounds of grain to produce one pound of edible animal meat and that animal is typically fed cash-crop imports that cause starvation in the developing world. The environmental think tank Worldwatch Institute explains that "the grain [fed to animals] would be used more efficiently [if] consumed directly by humans. Continued growth in meat output is dependent on feeding grain to animals, creating competition for grain between affluent meat eaters and the world's poor." Here again: if something is better for you, it's likely to be better all around. A plant-based diet reduces our dependence on a system of trade that harms the environment and the global poor. And that is good for everyone.

Some people will ask, "Won't a vegetarian diet require a lot more land to grow all that grain and all those vegetables?" You may laugh at the question, but I hear it rather often. It's an indication of just how little we think about how our food comes to us. The sad fact is that 83 percent of U.S. agricultural land is used for pasture or to grow crops to feed animals, to fatten them up so that we can eat them. Farmed animals are like us—most of what they eat simply sustains them; it doesn't go toward growth. So most of that corn, wheat, soy, and grain is wasted keeping farmed animals alive or growing their blood and bone, which we don't eat. Only a small fraction of it goes into creating flesh and fat for humans to eat— environmentally speaking, it is a huge waste to expend so much water and energy (and so many toxic fertilizers) on crops, only a fraction of which are actually turned into edible energy for humans.

Inefficiency is the least of it. Just recently, the United Nations published a report on livestock and the environment with a stunning conclusion: "The livestock sector emerges as one of the top two or three most significant contributors to the most serious environmental problems, at every scale from local to global." It turns out that raising animals for food is a primary cause of land degradation, air pollution, water shortage, water pollution, loss of biodiversity, and not least of all, global warming (or "climate crisis" or "climate change" as it is now called).

If you have your eyes and ears open, you can't help but hear the buzz about how emissions of greenhouse gases such as carbon dioxide are changing our climate, and scientists warn of more extreme weather, coastal flooding, spreading disease, and mass extinctions. The UN report says that almost a fifth of the emissions that contribute to global warming come from livestock (including chickens, pigs, and sheep in addition to cattle); more emissions than from all of the world's cars, trucks, and planes combined! In fact, a University of Chicago study determined that switching from a standard American diet to a vegan diet reduces greenhouse gas emissions more than switching from a regular car to a hybrid.

It gets even worse when we include the vast quantities of land needed to give us our chicken nuggets, steak, and pork chops. Animal agriculture takes up an incredible 70 percent of agricultural land worldwide; as a result, farmed animals are probably the biggest cause of the slashing and burning of the world's forests. Today, 70 percent of former Amazon rainforest is used for pastureland, and feed crops cover much of the remainder. These forests serve as "sinks," absorbing carbon dioxide from the air, and when the forests are burned all the stored carbon dioxide is released, in quantities that by far exceed the fossil fuel emissions of animal agriculture. As if that weren't bad enough, the real kicker comes when you look at gases besides carbon dioxide—gases like methane and nitrous oxide, enormously powerful greenhouse gases with an estimated 23 and 296 times the warming power of carbon dioxide, respectively.

If carbon dioxide is responsible for about one half of human-related greenhouse gas warming since the industrial revolution, methane and nitrous oxide are responsible for one-third. These super-strong gases come primarily from farmed animals' digestive processes and manure. Animal agriculture accounts for 9 percent of our carbon dioxide emissions, it emits 37 percent of our methane and a whopping 65 percent of our nitrous oxide.

It's all a bit hard to take in when you think of a small chick hatching from her fragile egg. How can an animal, so seemingly insignificant against the vastness of the earth, give off so much greenhouse gas as to change the global climate? The answer is in their sheer numbers.

With 10 billion land animals slaughtered every year to satisfy a meat-ravenous culture of half-pound steaks and all-you-can-eat buffets, it's hard to remember that not so long ago, meat was considered a luxury.

Land animals raised for food make up a staggering 20 percent of the entire land animal biomass of the earth. You could say that we are eating our planet to death. And what we are seeing is just the beginning. Meat consumption has increased fivefold in the past fifty years and is expected to double again in the next fifty.

Animal agriculture also accounts for most of the water consumed in this country, generates two-thirds of the world's acid-rain-causing ammonia, and is the world's largest source of water pollution—killing entire river and marine ecosystems, destroying coral reefs, and of course, making people sick. Try to imagine the prodigious volumes of manure churned out by modern American farms: 5 million tons a day, more than a hundred times that of the human population, and far more than our land can possibly absorb. The acres and acres of cesspools stretching over much of our countryside, polluting the air and contaminating our water make the *Exxon Valdez* oil spill look minor in comparison. We could address all this surprisingly easily by putting down our chicken wings and reaching for the faux chicken wings instead.

Conclusion

Some of us are obsessed with the numbers, the proteins and amino acids, the fats and carbs. But I'm certain that we were not put on this earth to be walking calculators or to maniacally study the scientific breakdown of our food before we ingest it. Of course it's good to become aware of what the body needs to fuel its health and to stay away from what bogs it down, but that should not be an obsessive focus. I would venture to guess that none of the great sages and thinkers of antiquity "counted calories." They ate to live, rather than living to eat.

Perhaps the more central task here is that we choose our food with spiritual integrity. What we eat should be good for our bodies as well as our souls. We can all accomplish a truly massive leap in wellness by staying alert and adhering to the great wisdom passed down through the ages that advises us to be loving, merciful, and compassionate.

Within those same spiritual doctrines we are warned against being greedy, gluttonous, or ignorant. It is prudent that we think about every aspect of how food arrives on our plate—how it's grown, how the workers who handle it are treated, how it is packaged, and how it is prepared. Eating with spiritual and moral integrity is far more important to our overall wellness than gauging carbohydrates and fat grams. Numerous studies show unequivocally that a plant-based diet is much healthier than a meat-based one. We can rejoice in losing weight and lowering our cholesterol, but at the end of the day how much love we are putting into the world and how much stress or suffering we are alleviating are the more significant measures.

As Buddhist writer Jeanne DuPrau writes in her lovely book *The Earth House,*

It isn't easy to turn around and start walking in the other direction on that road that can lead either toward or away from suffering, but we can practice for it in whatever small ways present themselves. We can transport spiders out of the path of danger, if we are willing to be thought mildly ridiculous; we can give over part of the vegetable garden to the gophers and the deer; we can stop shutting the lamb and the pig and the cow out of our imaginations, which will make us less and less interested in eating their legs and sides and rumps. We aren't going to achieve complete harmlessness, but we can take some steps in that direction. The point of saving all sentient beings is not to ensure the personal health and happiness of every bug, bird, fish, and animal on the planet. It is simply to foster the attitude that leads away from suffering. We can't change the world so that no one gets sick, no one is hurt, no one dies. The best we can do is take care of suffering where we find it. We save all beings because in the process of doing so we expand the boundaries of our identity; we push out the fences that limit what we can love.

Chapter Eight

One Bite at a Time
Assumptions and Truths, Questions and Answers About Eating Consciously

I'M NOT SUGGESTING THAT YOU BECOME VEGETARIAN OR VEGAN OVER-night. This is a hot issue and surely a sensitive one, with many layers to it. I resisted for a long time myself, so I understand. I am proposing this shift (or at least thoughtful consideration of it) because becoming vegan was probably the most profound change—on so many levels—I have ever made in my life. As I will discuss below, my energy level improved, but more critically, I continue to feel a daily joy at living according to my values. And I know from talking with and working with lots and lots of people, that I am far from alone.

One of the key points that I've been trying to make in this book is the need for conscious living. Meditation, cleansing, self analysis, exercise—it's all focused on one goal: living your life in a fully conscious way. The one suggestion that I have for you in that regard, one that actually requires no additional time at all, is to move toward a vegetarian or vegan diet, so that each time you eat, you'll be making a choice that rejects cruelty and oppression. Saint Paul counsels the Thessalonians to "pray without ceasing." One way to begin to make our lives a constant prayer is to make our daily routine, including eating, a statement of kindness. Albert Einstein summed up this concept when he wrote, "It is my view that the vegetarian manner of living by its purely physical effect on the human temperament would most beneficially influence the lot of mankind."

I also feel an obligation to expose the very real and tragic shadow of the current way of eating. If what I'm saying resonates with you, wonderful. If not, I respect your path entirely. Everyone has a unique physiology, individual needs, and is at a different place along the wellness continuum, so if you take from this discussion only the idea of "leaning into" conscious eating and giving a plant-based diet a little more consideration, I will have done my job. Should you decide to further implement some steps for going vegetarian, however, please read on and let me tell you a bit about how I made changes to my diet.

When I finally realized, however reluctantly, that I would have to take action, the first thing I did was make a list of all my trepidations about giving up meat and going vegetarian. I tried to apply my homegrown process of starting with awareness and *then* worrying about making the move. Even as I still ate meat and felt guilty about it, I trusted that if I was willing, I could make the change. This had worked for me with smoking, why not now?

But this was no small task for me, as I grew up loving southern fried chicken and turkey at Thanksgiving, ham at Christmas, and the cultural fun of hot dog and burger cookouts in the summertime. And even though I felt spiritually "called" to stop eating meat, I wasn't sure how to do it without jeopardizing my health.

Talking about what we *should* and *shouldn't* eat often brings up some very old and primal feelings. Food serves so many different functions for us: it connects us to family and cultural traditions; it brings us comfort, signals our prosperity, satisfies emotional, physical, and spiritual needs. But the more we learn about the ethical, health, and environmental impacts of our food choices, the more it seems obvious that it's time to confront our diets and make choices that truly support not only our bodies but the body of the world and all its inhabitants. Believe me, I know this is tough stuff.

When I first decided to transition to a vegetarian diet, I had many fears and, as it turned out, incorrect assumptions. I had a lot to learn. Let me share some of these with you so you can see what I mean.

Assumption: It's hard to be a vegetarian.

Truth: Being a vegetarian—or vegan, which means avoiding all animal products, including eggs, milk, or cheese—isn't difficult. You can surf around the Web and find tons of recipes and meal plans that are easy and inexpensive. These days a good number of fast-food places and chains offer veggie burgers. Most ethnic restaurants have many wonderful options. Much of my favorite food comes from Thai, Japanese, Middle Eastern, Greek, and Mexican restaurants, where I enjoy trying a wide variety of interesting dishes like tofu satay (grilled and served with a spicy peanut dipping sauce), hummus, bean burritos, and a vast array of salads. All major grocery stores carry soy milk and mock meats ("chicken" nuggets, barbeque "ribs," soy burgers, and soy sausage) and most even have vegan cheeses and soy ice cream. Some of these foods are extremely processed, so you probably won't want to live on them, but they're better than the foods they replace, and they're good in a pinch, especially as you lean away from meat. Again, it's all about upgrading your choices gradually and comfortably. If you can't find what you want at your local store, the management will most likely order it for you. And there is nothing more colorful and seasonable than a farmers market on the weekend!

When going to a friend's house for dinner, you can just say, "Don't bother getting a steak or piece of fish for me, because I'm vegetarian; I would be happy to bring a veggie burger to throw on the grill so you don't have to go out of your way for me." So far, in my experience, no one has taken offense at that, and if anything, my veganism becomes an interesting topic of conversation.

As for maintaining what I thought would be a very strict and difficult discipline, it took me only a few weeks to get used to the changes in my diet. I eased myself off meat and dairy products gradually, so it wasn't like I suddenly found myself in completely new territory without all the creature comforts (excuse the pun!). It is so much easier to do things bit by bit so you don't overwhelm your system and go back to your old ways. I learned what was easy to make (salads, stir fry, rice and beans) and made sure I never felt deprived. The hardest thing for me to give up was café latte; it was my absolute favorite indulgence (that and hot milk and honey before I went to bed). But I'd heard that it takes about twenty-one days to change your taste buds, so I just kept ordering soy lattes even though I didn't like them, hoping that eventually I would get used to the taste. And in fact that is exactly what happened. I travel a lot, and a big issue for me is having good food on the road. You can find oatmeal for breakfast in almost any diner or hotel restaurant. I bring a stash of almonds and walnuts with me and sprinkle them on top with some blueberries or a banana and it always satisfies me. I also bring prepackaged protein powder and shake it up in a bottle of water for when I need an extra boost. For lunch or dinner, there are always salads, potatoes (yams are even better), avocados, and vegetables to be found. And if I am in any sort of city, I always run to the local health food store to see what they have to offer; I enjoy seeing what I can find that is local to that area. If I am making a day trip, I'll whip up a sandwich before leaving the house with tomatoes, sprouts, vegetarian slices of "meat" and "cheese" and whatever else I can throw into the pita or whole grain bread. It's also really important to eat fresh fruits and vegetables, so I bring some prewashed cut-up broccoli and an apple to eat throughout the day.

Assumption: Well, I can just shop for humane, organic, or kosher meat knowing that at least the animals were treated better.

Truth: Sadly, most of the meat, egg, and dairy companies that pretend to be eco- or animal-friendly, with packages covered in pictures of pretty red barnyards, are the same massive, corporately owned factory farms.

Labels like "Swine Welfare" and "UEP Certified" are simply the industry labels (the "Swine Welfare" label comes from the National Pork Producers Council and the UEP stands for the United Egg Producers; both are trade groups that exist only to maximize profits, and their explanations for their labels are filled with grandiose rhetoric, which doesn't do much good for the animals). The labels hide what really happens behind closed doors as animals are turned into meat for our tables.

As the demand for organic food grows, industrial farms are increasingly switching to an organic system in a way that violates the spirit, and sometimes even the letter, of what it means to be organic. (The animal welfare regulations for USDA-approved organic farms are exceedingly weak.) And unfortunately, "kosher" does not live up to its original intent when it comes to how animals are treated on farms, and the largest kosher slaughterhouse in North America was caught horribly abusing animals—ripping the tracheae out of live cows' throats and worse—and defending the abuse as kosher. A video download documenting the abuse is listed in the index, and Rabbi Michael Lerner, founder of *Tikkun*, calls watching it "a moral imperative for anyone who eats meat."

All that said, the meat eater who limits him or herself to grass-fed cattle flesh is making a much smaller negative impact than most other meat eaters. If you have decided that you want to go vegetarian but simply can't give up all meat, far and away the least-cruel animal product is grass-fed cattle.

Assumption: Vegetarians sometimes seem preachy, judgmental, or extreme.

Truth: Some of us are, but most of us are not; it's just that the loud ones make the headlines and get the attention. I asked a longtime vegetarian friend about this, and I think his theory is probably right. He believes that some new vegetarians are so horrified by what they learn that they feel duty bound to bludgeon everyone they can find into "seeing the light," sort of like some religious fundamentalists. The veggie zealots either mellow or burn out, because you can't sustain that level of anger about a problem so intractable. Of course, that doesn't mean the damage hasn't already been done: these folks do manage to alienate a fair number of people before they tone down or go away.

Assumption: There must be some people for whom vegetarian food is not an option.

Truth: This is the case if you are living in the Arctic or in sub-Saharan Africa. If you are born into or live in a place and situation where there is no choice, you certainly have to make the best of what is available. That said, most of us really do have options. Many of the alternatives available now weren't around even ten years ago; it has never been easier to take the steps toward being vegetarian.

As for food allergies or sensitivities, a good nutritionist (or a nutrition-oriented book) will be able to help you make safe choices. It may sound trite but it's true: if you have a will to eat consciously, a way to do it will become apparent. It may not be the easiest path, but most people who travel it will testify that it is both easy and fun. And becoming healthy and conscious is worth the time and effort you put into it; I guarantee you will feel cleaner and clearer—sort of like being at the vortex of life—when you work out a system that is both health giving and soul nurturing. In any case, as long as you are thinking about it and desiring to become ever more aware and compassionate, you are well on your way to a stepped up new version of yourself.

Assumption: Since humans have always eaten animals, maybe that is just the natural order of things.

Truth: Actually, like those of most herbivores, almost all our teeth are flat and blunt, including our incisors. As the renowned anthropologist Dr. Richard Leakey says, "You can't tear flesh by hand, you can't tear hide by hand. . . . We wouldn't have been able to deal with food sources that required those large canines." Our hands are rather good for grabbing and picking fruits and vegetables though! And also, like the intestines of other herbivores, ours are very long (carnivores have short intestines so they can quickly get rid of all that rotting flesh they eat). We don't have sharp claws to seize and hold down prey. And most of us I hope lack the instinct that would drive us to chase and then kill animals and devour their raw carcasses. If you want to learn more about the physiologies associated with different diets, Dr. Milton Mills, of the Physicians' Committee for Responsible Medicine, has written an excellent essay called "The Comparative Anatomy of Eating." We may be omnivores in that we *can* survive on just about anything, but that doesn't mean that we shouldn't think about making food choices that are responsible, kind, and healthy. See the Suggested Reading and Viewing section at the end of this book.

The point is, thousands of years ago, when we were hunter-gatherers, we may have needed a bit of meat in our diets in times of scarcity, but we don't need it now. William C. Roberts, M.D., editor of the *American Journal of Cardiology*, says, "Although we think we are, and we act as if we are, human beings are not natural carnivores. When we kill animals to eat them, they end up killing us, because their flesh, which contains cholesterol and saturated fat, was never intended for human beings, who are natural herbivores."

If you are not moved by the spiritual arguments against eating meat, just remember that our evolution in human morality is marked almost entirely by our attempt to move beyond the "might makes right" law of the jungle. It may indeed be "natural" for the powerful to dominate the weak, but that doesn't mean it's the right way to be. We have become better informed and hopefully more conscious over the eons; we have more choices and options now than ever before. Perhaps our dominion over animals does not mean that we should be able to do anything we want with them, but rather that we are charged to look after them, making sure that we treat them fairly and with the same compassion we afford every creation of Spirit.

Assumption: Might this be a slippery slope? If I give up eating meat, what about leather? Or wool? Or meat-based dog food? Am I now to start worrying about not killing insects, too? Aren't plants living also? Where do I draw the line?

Truth: Of course, the fact that we can't do everything should not mean that we then choose to do nothing. Remember, we are on a continuum. Progress, not perfection! We may indeed decide to do more or go further in our endeavors to be conscientious as time goes by, but we need not refuse to be kind *now* for fear that we might have to be kinder still.

Regarding plants, the Christian writer C. S. Lewis staunchly opposed testing on animals on scriptural grounds, and to those who asked whether there is a difference between cruelty to animals and cruelty to plants, he pointed out that people already understand the differences. Each of us would recoil in horror if asked to imagine an animal being bludgeoned or dismembered alive—because we know that these things cause animals pain. We can see it, feel it, and empathize. But none of us feels similarly at the prospect of pulling weeds or breaking up a head of lettuce or mowing our lawn—because we know both intuitively and from scientific studies that weeds and lawns and heads of lettuce can't feel pain.

I'll admit that I am surprised by how often someone will argue that there is no difference between eating plants and eating animals—because plants are alive. But plants don't have any of the things that are required to feel pain—a central nervous system, a brain, pain receptors. As an aside, it takes a lot more plants to feed the animals we eat than it takes to feed us directly. So if you're worried about plant pain, you'll save exponentially more plants by eating them yourself, rather than funneling them through animals.

I'm not so sure about insects, though I try to give them the benefit of the doubt whenever possible. Yes, when I walk down the street, I'm sure I step on bugs. But then we have to ask ourselves, does the fact that we can't stop all pain mean that we shouldn't bother to stop a lot of it? Of course not. That would be like saying that if you drive a car, you shouldn't even bother to recycle, or that since I accidentally step on some bugs, I shouldn't step around the ones I happen to notice. We do what we can to be kind within the context of living a normal and healthy, nonobsessive life.

There are those who may ask goading questions, such as "If you were on a desert island and it was just you and a pig, would you eat the pig?" or "If a building were on fire and there were a baby and a chicken, which would you save?" Of course I'd eat the pig. Of course I'd save the baby. The thing about vegetarianism is that there is no real trade-off: eating meat—in almost every way you look at it—is not good for us. By giving it up, you are sparing animals horrible suffering and pain, and all you are giving up is a few potentially enjoyable meals. In the long run, both you and the animal will benefit.

Now the questions get more difficult to answer. It took me years to give up leather, because frankly I was far more attached to my shoes than I was to my steak dinner. But the more I thought about it, the less comfortable I felt about buying leather. I came to understand many shocking realities. Much leather is imported from India and China, where spent dairy cows who are so totally broken and withered that they cannot be used for flesh are used only for leather. I watched a horrible video of emaciated animals piled on top of each other in trucks on the way to slaughter. They were slaughtered with dull blades and skinned before they were even dead. The video also made the point that leather decomposes unless it's thoroughly treated with toxic chemicals, and since most leather comes from developing countries with no enforced worker or environmental protection regulations, the workers in these factories are touching and breathing in the chemicals all day long; and then the used chemicals are dumped into rivers, turning them to toxic sludge.

Leather, like meat, is terrible for the environment and the workers who put leather goods together, and even if something is assembled ("made") in Italy (or wherever), most of the raw material comes from China or India. Even knowing all this, I still kept buying leather products for a long time, but I gradually weaned myself from them and started looking for canvas and faux-leather alternatives (still not great for the environment, but a lot better than leather). I have found several great designers who make shoes and bags without leather, and interestingly, the cheapest accessories are nonleather anyway, so I'm saving a lot of money! I've also made a sort of sport of finding leather alternatives and take great satisfaction in knowing that I satisfied my shopping cravings without hurting anyone.

As for wool, dog and cat food, and the like, I see this awakening to conscious consumption as a progression. We can't do everything at once, and it is a process of unfolding. To change everything with one fell swoop would be such a shock that it would be all too tempting to go back to sleep (to our old ways of eating and purchasing) when things got too difficult or overwhelming.

One step at a time, one choice upgraded after another, until we find ourselves moving jauntily along our path of all-around wellness. And then, as with all things quantum, suddenly you find yourself living at a new level with hardly a disruption at all.

Assumption: Being vegetarian is good enough. Vegans are going overboard!

Question: What is the difference between vegetarian and vegan?

Truth: Being vegetarian means that you don't eat any animals—no beef, chicken, pork, lamb, or fish; being vegan means eating no animal *products* at all, including dairy and eggs. I was vegetarian for a long time before I became vegan. I thought I needed the calcium from milk and figured it would be way too hard to give up my favorite cheeses and omelets. To be vegan sounded extreme to me, so I just put that on the back burner and satisfied myself with knowing that at least I wasn't eating actual animals.

Then a friend explained that dairy cows are lactating females who give birth to one baby per year to keep their milk flowing. When male calves are born (about a million each year), they are shipped to veal farms. The veal industry originated in "America's Dairyland," as a cruel but convenient answer to the problem of surplus male calves. The veal and dairy industries work in a sad symbiosis.

The moment they are born, veal calves (babies!) are ripped away from their mothers, all the while mooing furiously for her as she tries to follow, and confined (often with their necks chained) to a crate barely bigger than their bodies (22 by 58 inches) so that they can hardly turn around or lie down; this causes their muscles to atrophy and remain tender. For four months—the time they have on this earth until slaughter—they generally live in the dark without ever getting to suckle, play in the field, learn to walk on their wobbly legs, or do anything else but stew in their own filth. They are denied solid food to chew on and made anemic (they lick ravenously at the metal chain to get the iron that a growing calf instinctively craves) so that their flesh stays a pale white. When they are sold at auction by dairy farmers, before being shipped to slaughter, they sometimes cannot walk and are therefore dragged. If you've ever seen a baby calf, it would break your heart to know that this innocent little creature (cattle are very gentle and affectionate by nature) must endure such an awful fate as to be designated veal.

In fact I already knew about veal and had stayed away from it for a very long time. But when I realized that by eating dairy products I was supporting the veal industry, it only made sense to stop. The same principles hold true regarding eggs. I was shocked to learn that the cruelest of the common factory-farmed products are eggs (foie gras is in its own category, but since most people don't eat it, I'll spare you; Google it if you want to find out more—the videos will blow your mind, and break your heart). Egg-laying hens are packed tightly together into battery cages that measure about 18 by 20 inches. Since their typical wingspan is 30 inches, you can imagine how maddeningly painful it must be to share the cage with four to eight other birds who also can't move.

Because chickens who are caged cannot satisfy their natural pecking instincts, they turn on each other in what can only be understood as severe frustration and panic—like any living creature would, crammed into such close confines, for their entire lives. So the egg industry has determined that cutting off the ends of their beaks (without anesthesia) sufficiently prevents them from damaging each other—or the company's bottom line. According to scientists, the process, which the industry recently decided to call (in an unintentional nod to George Orwell) "beak trimming" (it used to be called debeaking) causes severe pain that lasts for more than a month. They are housed by the tens of thousands in filthy sheds, and what's worse, the baby male chicks who serve no purpose (they can't lay eggs and are of a different strain from meat chickens) are ground up alive and disposed of.

As for my concern about getting enough calcium if I gave up dairy, it turns out that you can get the calcium you need from certain green leafy vegetables, almonds, or even fortified soy or rice milk. And regarding the high protein I thought I was getting from eggs, it appears that eggs have the same arachidonic acid—the inflammatory compound that may have a lot to do with cancer and heart disease—as do the chickens themselves, so they are best avoided as well.

In fact, eggs may be one of the most unhealthy foods around; the rates of salmonella contamination are frightening, and every egg contains as much artery-clogging cholesterol (210 to 225 milligrams of cholesterol per egg) as three servings of beef (three ounces of beef contains 60 to 80 milligrams of cholesterol)! Once again, it seems that what is good for our health is also good for our humanity.

Assumption: Slaughterhouses may be awful, but at least these places provide jobs to people.

Truth: Actually, the workers are treated so badly that in a major report called "Blood, Sweat, and Fear: Workers' Rights in U.S. Meat and Poultry Plants," Human Rights Watch called slaughterhouse worker treatment in the United States a human rights violation. It's common for factory farms to have an extremely high turnover of laborers in a single year. The injury rates and working conditions are abominable. Human Rights Watch calls slaughterhouse work the "most dangerous factory job in America." If workers who really need a job in the worst way can hardly bear to stay for more than a year, one has to wonder why anyone would want to *eat* the product of what happens in one of these hellish places.

Becoming a vegetarian or vegan is enormously empowering. It's about having integrity in the most fundamental of all our actions—eating. When we have integrity, we grow in compassion and consciousness. We discover just how connected everything really is: what is good for our physical health is also good for our spiritual and emotional well-being and for the global community and environment of which we are a part.

Notable thinkers from Leonardo da Vinci to Albert Schweitzer to Mohandas Gandhi to Leo Tolstoy have argued that if our every meal is based on support for violence and cruelty, we will inevitably also have wars and daily violence, and that if our meals are based in compassion, we will be far less likely to support wars and daily violence. The great thinker and mathematician Pythagoras (vegetarians were often called Pythagoreans until the term *vegetarian* arose, in the nineteenth century) stated that, "As long as humanity continues to be the ruthless destroyer of lower living beings, he will never know health or peace. For as long as men massacre animals, they will kill each other. Indeed, he who sows the seed of murder and pain cannot reap joy and love."

Making the Transition

So now that you know that a plant-based diet is a good choice for the planet, your health, and animals, you may wonder how to start making the transition to a diet that is more in keeping with your values. If you have been eating meat your whole life, as I had been, this sort of a change can seem daunting. Happily, it's easier than ever to switch to a vegetarian or vegan diet, and you don't have to do it all at once. In fact, the following suggestions should help even the most die-hard carnivores make the switch.

The thing to remember throughout your process—with this or any other self-improvement endeavor—is that once you set your intention to upgrade, you've already started the wheels in motion. Just keep taking baby steps and leaning into being the person you want to be. Continue to keep your eyes and your heart open, letting new information settle in and affect you. Remain willing to change, even if you aren't moved to do so right at this moment. Then, make the incremental shifts in as many areas as you feel comfortable. Push yourself ever so slightly beyond your comfort zone. And before you know it, a radical (yet gentle!) change will have occurred. Here we go:

1. **If you are not yet ready to give up meat altogether, start by eating meatless meals one or two days a week.** The Johns Hopkins School of Public Health, Columbia University's School of Public Health, and other public-health schools have designed a "Meatless Monday" campaign to help people avoid our four top killers: heart disease, stroke, diabetes, and cancer—by eating meat-free at least every Monday. The "Meatless Monday" program provides recipes, meal plans, nutritional guidelines, cooking tips, and more. I wish the campaign also steered people away from fish, because fish are definitely not vegetables, but it's certainly a good start.

2. Give up the little animals first. Although many people tend to stop eating red meat before they give up chicken, turkey, or fish, from a humane standpoint, this is backward. Birds are arguably the most abused animals on the planet, and birds and fish yield less flesh than cows or pigs, so commercial farmers and fisheries kill more of them to satisfy America's meat habit. If you choose to give up meat in stages, I'd suggest that you stop eating chickens and turkeys first, and then fish, and then pigs and cows. In fact, you'll be helping animals more by giving up eggs than beef; ten times as many animals are killed by the egg industry as the beef industry, and the egg industry is even worse than the veal industry on the cruelty scale.

From an environmental standpoint, some will suggest that cattle are the worst for the environment because they contribute more greenhouse gases, but that seems like hairsplitting to me. After all, the Amazon rainforest is now being cut down to grow soybeans to feed chickens; it's chicken and pig farms that are poisoning the Atlantic Ocean, and vastly more energy is required if we eat the chickens who are fed grain rather than eating that grain directly.

3. If you can't give up one particular animal product, give up all the other ones. One friend of mine told me that he just loves burgers too much to stop eating them; I suggested that he give up all animal products except burgers. Some of my friends can't (or won't) give up ice cream or cream in their coffee—so I say give up everything but that. That is a huge step forward, and I suspect that after eating mostly vegetarian for a while, you'll decide that those burgers or that ice cream aren't so tasty anymore. And you will probably find that you enjoy the faux meats and dairy-free options just as much.

4. Examine your diet and begin to substitute. Take a look at the meals that you and your family already enjoy, and you will probably notice that many of them can be made without any meat or with mock meats (which are great transition foods) instead of animal flesh. For example, instead of spaghetti and meat sauce, make spaghetti and marinara sauce (and if you crumble tofu into it, I dare say no one will suspect that it isn't beef, because tofu takes on the taste of the sauce); instead of beef burritos, try bean burritos. Or you can replace the ground beef with the vegetarian variety, which can be found in just about any grocery store. There are many websites (several are listed at the back of this book) that will assist you in finding products to fill out your shopping list. Mock meats, nondairy cheeses and milks, and other vegetarian foods are sold in most major supermarkets these days, and health food stores offer even more.

There are excellent soy creamers, and even the most mainstream coffeehouses offer a nondairy alternative. And if you like to bake, look for egg replacer, a powdered mix of natural ingredients like potato starch that can be used instead of eggs in cakes and other baked goods (or you can just use applesauce). Most importantly though, don't forget to eat your vegetables—as well as plenty of whole grains, fresh fruits, and legumes—instead of filling up on cake and carbohydrate-laden treats.

After a few meatless meals, you will likely realize that you don't even miss meat and are ready to go meatless for good. But don't beat yourself up if you slip every now and again; before long, eating vegetarian will come as naturally as breathing.

I know that some of you who are already vegetarian might take issue with the idea of relying on faux meats; they are indeed more processed and less of a whole food. But mock meats and soy milk are superb transition foods and will help you to feel less deprived. You can gradually move into a diet made up solely of grains, beans, vegetables, and fruits; but go at a comfortable pace. Veggie burgers, "hot dogs," "chicken" nuggets, and so on, are healthy choices, providing healthy plant protein without any of the cholesterol or saturated animal fats found in meat. Whichever vegetarian foods you choose, animals and your sense of spiritual integrity will benefit.

5. **Eat out thoughtfully.** Countless restaurants cater to vegetarians and vegans, and there are many regional restaurants and restaurant chains that offer vegetarian options. If they don't, you can request that the chef do an interesting vegetable plate. I always ask for something with lots of fresh vegetables and some legumes if they have them. A baked potato or artichoke with olive oil is also good to add into the mix.

6. **But "don't sweat the small stuff."** Vegans and vegan wannabes shouldn't be too concerned about ingredients that make up less than two percent of their meal. You will obviously want to avoid dishes served with meat, cheese, or eggs, but you need not get crazy if there is a dab of butter or whey or other animal product in the bun your veggie burger is served on. You won't appreciably stop animal suffering by avoiding such minuscule amounts of animal ingredients. The goal is to eat in a conscious, animal-friendly manner without driving friends, family, or the waiters at restaurants nuts.

If you are wondering why I've spent such a great deal of time focusing on eating consciously, it's because it is the single most fundamental and simple thing you can do to create the most far-reaching and monumental shift. It is a shortcut to quantum wellness in every sense of the term. When you consider your choices—heart disease, cancer, plus-size pants, melting ice caps, gale-force storms, and animal suffering versus good health, abundant energy, a trim physique, a livable planet, compassion, and tasty diverse foods—it is clear that going vegetarian is an excellent choice as we move toward living a more conscious life. And we can do this one step at a time.

We are on a path, not a race; although I will say that in recent years the need for change has become more urgent. But even as much as we should push ourselves past old limitations so that the breakthroughs can begin, we can also allow ourselves the room to make the changes at a pace that will likely result in permanent change.

Try this:

1. Start by eating just one meatless meal per week and build from there.

2. Give up the little animals first: chickens and turkeys first, then fish, then pigs and cows. In fact, you'll be helping more animals by giving up eggs than by giving up beef.

3. If there's one meat product you can't give up, like bacon or steak, give up all the others.

4. Look around for substitutions. They're everywhere, and they taste really good!

5. If you're going out to eat, order the vegetarian option. If they don't have one, ask, ask, and keep asking. Almost any restaurant can come up with something to serve you. Plus, if we all keep asking, pretty soon all food service providers—restaurants, hotels, corporate cafeterias, etc.—will get the hint and add better options to their menus.

CHAPTER NINE

Personal Energy Management
Balancing the Four Rs

BY NOW YOU'VE GOT SOME POWERFUL PRACTICES FOR HANDLING PAIN, stress, and mental chatter, for cleansing your body and creating a nest where you feel at your creative best, and now for eating in a way that fully supports your wellness. But all this will be for naught if you can't find balance in your life.

For many of us, the biggest issue is time. We don't know how to prioritize, and we find a zillion pressing reasons to justify not taking the time to care for ourselves on all the levels that make us well-integrated, healthy human beings. But we'll never experience quantum wellness if we keep letting the world sap us dry. We have to decide where to put our energy and ration ourselves according to our deepest values. It doesn't matter what we *say* is most important, it's where we place the bulk of our energy that speaks to who we really are.

Look at how you spend your days and you will see what your priorities are. Most of us are imbalanced in one way or another; we obsess over our kids, or we addictively try to get ahead with work. Some of us get wrapped up in our emotional dramas while others get lost in shopping trips and socializing. We can't just leave our energy free to roam at will or it will just fall into whatever is crying the loudest for our attention. No, if we want a grander and more glorious experience of being alive, we have to recognize the choices we are making and make better ones! Yes, it's as simple as that.

I have found the following quadrant model extremely useful in analyzing how I use my energy. Keeping a balance between the four Rs will bring your life into equilibrium and help you maintain forward momentum in your quest for quantum wellness. I'm not suggesting scheduling every minute of your day, but rather making a practice of simply checking in from time to time to make sure you are dipping into all the quadrants. Reminding yourself of the four categories will ensure that you don't get lost or overly focused in one area while letting the others fall by the wayside.

The **regular** quadrant covers everything that is part of your everyday routine, your set obligations. This is where we spend most of our time. There's always more to do. You have to walk the dog, feed the kids, get to the grocery store, and prepare the report. There are business meetings and taxes to pay and things to fix when they break. The house needs cleaning and the car needs an oil change and there are calls and e-mails to catch up on. If you spend all your time in the regular quadrant, you'll be fooled into thinking that life is only about keeping your head above water. Of course, the paradox here is that the more you do, the more you can find that is still undone.

People who get lost in this section are often perfectionists; they can't walk into a room without seeing something askew and then addressing it. Their lives are filled with lists and they wake up in the middle of the night gripped by panic at the thought of what they forgot to accomplish or didn't do correctly. If this rings a bell with you, then know that too much of your energy is being spent on simply trying to keep up.

It's tempting to stick to what you know and not stretch yourself, because there is comfort in repetition. You know how to run the house or work at your job. You can clean out the garage and get a sense of accomplishment. That's great. But if you fill up all your time with this routine stuff, you will have missed out on so much of life.

So get your regular list taken care of, but don't worry about dotting every *i* or crossing each *t*. Go at it with the sense that you will give it your full attention until you've done enough for the day. You'll know that it's enough when you start really considering the other areas as equally important to your wellness. As you become more aware and conscientious of your integral well-being, you will sense a click of completion when it's time to redirect your energy to one of the other Rs.

On the flip side, if you are someone who *avoids* taking responsibility for the basics—you just can't seem to get around to paying your bills or shopping for some healthy food—it's time to start spending more time in this quadrant. Get out a pad of paper and write down everything that absolutely must get done. Now shave off some time from the other categories and start ticking off the items on that list. Start with the easiest and most doable things; finishing them will give you a sense of accomplishment. Clean the kitchen, open the mail, and do a load of laundry. Once those things are done, move it up a notch to things that are more involved: clear up your credit cards, make that difficult phone call you've been putting off, and respond to an e-mail that has been nagging at you. Once these things are firmly addressed, your energy will be freed up to take on more exciting projects.

Put your other endeavors—acting classes or all-consuming relationships, for instance—on the back burner until you bring up your energy in this most fundamental arena.

The **relate** quadrant covers more ground than you might expect. Our lives are all about relating to one another: to our partners, our kids, our friends, the store clerk, the boss, the board, etc. We are in near-constant contact with other people, learning to live together, negotiating our desires, and working through conflicts. We have ample opportunities to either lift each other up or make each other miserable, so this is an important area to be conscientious in. If you are wondering what relating has to do with wellness, think about how good you feel after being with certain people while with others your energy seems drained and depressed.

How we are in relationships and with whom very directly affects our outlook and sense of well-being. You can eat all the right things, exercise, and visualize all day long, but if you can't relate to others in a healthy way—in serious relationships as well as in brief encounters—you will never be a well-integrated, healthy and happy person. Throughout our lives we are given lessons to improve our skills at navigating interpersonal relationships, and with each conflict we bump up against, we are challenged to rise to our highest potential.

We are wired to become increasingly conscious and enlightened; you can tell this because it literally feels bad in your body when you've been unkind. I know if I've been short with someone, I get a cramped feeling in my chest or feel nauseated. If I disrespect some-one, I feel myself breathing shallowly and anxiety seems to race through my body until I right the wrong. Our bodies cue us to rise above our baser instincts. In the same way, when I deal with a con-flict successfully or act in a more conscious way in a situation that I had before not done well in, my energy seems to soar and I feel tri-umphant. I have twice the vigor when I'm doing right by my inner compass of principles and ethics.

Relationships, rife as they are with joys, disputes, and challenges, give us some of our best opportunities to evolve, and getting an accu-rate picture of how we perceive and react to people really shows us where we are on our continuum of growth and development.

If, for instance, you often find yourself grumbling with com-plaints or judgments about people in various areas of your life (you think your lawyer is not representing you well, your spouse is bor-ing and annoying, and the computer technician working on your lap-top is inept) you might consider that this sour outlook is more about what's going on inside of you rather than the shortcomings of those about whom you are complaining. After all, you are the common de-nominator. Of course there will always be people who do indeed fall short of their promises, but when there is a trend or a repetitive pat-tern (people are always letting you down or more often than not, you experience high drama), it would be wise to look closely at what en-ergy might be coming *from you* and is being mirrored back to you.

It is true, even if a bit cliché by now, that if there is negative en-ergy within us, we create negative energy, because just as water seeks its own level, like feels comfortable with like. We gravitate toward the familiar. If you want to feel more alive and become more vital and vibrant, look to how you operate in relationships and be-gin the work there. Notice how you affect people, and make it your business to be more authentic, kind, and open.

As you shift the way you relate (some of us need to work on stronger boundaries while others of us need to risk being intimate), your sense of well-being will also shift. Start with yourself. Become more honest with yourself and people will have straightforward conversations with you. Be more loving toward yourself, and others will follow suit. Soften in your attitudes and the world will cozy up to you. If you want to feel more comfortable and happy, work on making the people around you more comfortable and happy.

The person standing right in front of you at any given moment is the perfect person to start experimenting with. It isn't just the "big" relationships that count. You may want to consider that there just may be a divine design within every single interaction with every single person (or situation or even animal) that crosses your path.

Everything in this life is intricately interconnected to everything else, and each action you take, every word you say, alters the next moment that follows. Every encounter with another being is an opportunity to be respectful of the forces of nature that design our universe.

So, practice being responsible with your words and actions; learn to be more intimate and authentic; observe healthy boundaries; and finally, make amends where necessary and do better the next time around.

Whether or not you rise to that opportunity is entirely up to you. In the relate quadrant, the goal is to upgrade your behavior. There is always a gift in each relationship, be it casual or serious. Sometimes the gift is that you get to implement new behaviors or traits, and at other times the gift is that you can practice aligning your consciousness and values in a way that helps you become more in tune with the underlying Oneness that connects us all.

And please remember this: there is no one person on this earth who is any more valuable than any other. We all breathe the same air and each of us is working on our development in our own personal ways. Human beings are, genetically speaking, 99.9 percent identical. Even most animals share the majority of our genes. Someone's status, wealth, and accomplishments may entice you into believing that he is more or less important, but the truth is that we are, none of us, any better or worse than anyone else. We cross each other's paths for a reason, whether as an opportunity to learn something new or heal something old and woe begotten. In Tibetan Buddhism, it is said that every person at one point in time has been everything to you and vice versa. In other words, we have been each other's mother, sister, husband, jailer, employer, savior, and crucifier. They caution that the beggar you might be tempted to snub could have been your father in another life, or the criminal you dismiss as hopeless might have been the doctor who saved your child in the last go around. Whether or not you buy into the idea of life after life, the point is that you never know the full story of the person who stands in front of you. Treat him as if he is an angel in disguise, because he just might be.

This concept is well established in Judaism and Christianity, of course. Welcoming the stranger is a central Jewish injunction, and one can fulfill it even on the Sabbath. And who can forget Jesus's beautiful parable in Matthew 25, in which the central test of salvation is presented as whether one fed the hungry, welcomed the stranger, clothed the naked, and visited the sick and imprisoned?

Lord, when did we see you hungry and feed you, or thirsty and give you drink? When did we see you a stranger and welcome you, or naked and clothe you? When did we see you ill or in prison, and visit you? And in reply, Amen, I say to you, whatever you did for one of these least brothers of mine, you did for me. (Matthew 25: 37–40, New American Bible).

The task before each of us is to work on our communication skills, our ability to be kind and forgiving, and to open ourselves to the lessons and gifts offered to us by each and every person who comes into our life. If, though, you are overindulging in the relate quadrant (perhaps you spend too much time keeping up with friends or get your self-esteem only from being helpful), you will know it, because you'll have hardly any time or focus left over to tend to other things (like exercise or creativity). If this is the case, pull back a little energy for yourself, screen your phone calls, and allow people the space to live their lives without depending on you.

A life lived fully takes effort: you are taking care of business, handling obligations, maintaining your relationships, and trying to be an overall better person. You put a lot of energy out into the world, but you also need to rest and receive in order to strike a balance. In yoga, every active posture is followed by a position of rest so that the body-mind can freely and fully exert itself knowing that rest is soon to follow.

For many of us, self-care is one of the hardest things to do. Some of us feel guilty for taking time for "me," while others of us pack our schedules too tightly to allow ourselves the necessary downtime. But **rejuvenation**, in the long run, is not optional. Just as a car needs to be gassed up or the fridge needs restocking, if you want to keep going, you have to restore your reserves.

Many of us unwittingly neglect ourselves, putting off our needs until some future date when we will at last have some time. We're afraid that no one can do the job as well as we can or that if we let up the pressure even a little, everything will fall apart. But the truth is that if you push too hard for too long without rest, things will break down. We don't do anyone any favors by not resting when we're tired or not taking time to do things just for ourselves; rather, we become more tightly wound and even embittered or resentful. Not a pleasure to be around. Your relationships, your health, your ability to be creative—all will be greatly diminished if you don't take care of yourself.

Nourished people, people who love and care for themselves, are also more efficient and nicer to be around. When you give yourself permission to relax, people will feel more relaxed around you; your environment will become more harmonious. Balance—between work and pleasure, giving and receiving, seriousness and levity—creates a happy healthy life.

There's no one right way to rejuvenate; we each relax in different ways and have our own rhythms. We all need private time, friends, fun activities, love, and quiet. If you are an introvert like me, regular rejuvenation looks a little like this: I wake up slowly and quietly; I don't chat until after I've had my tea and breakfast and had ample time to read the paper. I go on a beautiful hike by myself or with a good friend at least several times a week. I don't book myself up with too many social engagements, because although I enjoy the company, I know I'll lose my grounding if I'm out too much. Even though I work very hard, I've chosen a career path that enables me to be in my own space, spend time with my dogs, and enjoy a good deal of quiet contemplation. I cherish the space that I've created for myself and it makes me feel very happy and vital.

My friend Harry, on the other hand, feels completely restored if he goes to a fun party or attends a lively concert. He likes action, and if he has too much quiet time he feels sluggish and out of touch. I remember recently he was coming down with a cold or flu and decided, against popular wisdom, that he needed to get out and socialize. For me, going out on the town would push me over the edge because it would wear me out. But because my friend is, for the most part, an extrovert, the buzz and excitement rejuvenated him and he went home with nary a symptom left. Extroverts need more activity; they refuel by being around people and in the center of things.

Whether you lean toward being an introvert or an extrovert, it's important to understand and cater to your nature so that you aren't trying to be something you're not. For instance, going to an amusement park is not fun for me; there is too much stimulation, and rather than feeling refueled, I feel exhausted at the end of the day. In much the same way, my friend Harry would not thrive at a week-long meditation retreat, because he would be bored to tears. He would be much better off going on an adventurous trip with a couple of guy friends.

Of course, if you are an extrovert in a relationship with an introvert, you can find ways to meet in the middle: exploring a new city together or having small dinner parties with friends, for example. The important thing is that you honor your needs and desires and listen to your inner voice when it's telling you to slow down (or get going).

Ask yourself what you need to do to take care of yourself today, at this moment. Regularly carve out a piece of your schedule to do things that make you feel good and rejuvenated. Don't wait until your work is done; stop for a few minutes or a few hours, or take a vacation. Give yourself a break. Relax without guilt and enjoy yourself knowing that to be truly well, balance is key.

On the other hand, if you think you are spending too much time rejuvenating—you can't tear yourself away from the poolside or say no to another shopping trip, for instance—you might want to remind yourself again that your life has purpose to it and in order to fulfill that purpose of growing and becoming a richer human being, some effort is required. Look at the graph and figure out how you can put time and energy into the other quadrants. Allow yourself only your budgeted amount of time to lollygag around, and schedule the rest of your day so that you don't have the opportunity to slip back into vacation mode. Nature abhors a vacuum, as they say; so fill in the time slots yourself, with purposeful action, until you get a momentum going.

Reach: In order to transcend your current state and move into quantum wellness, the inclination to remain status quo must be overcome. That's where the final quadrant comes in. It's one of the easiest areas to neglect, and it's so important not to.

Reaching is about conscientiously stretching yourself past what is habitual and comfortable. You take care of what needs to get done (regular), you tend to your relationships (relate), you nurture yourself and rest (rejuvenate), and then you take a deep breath and challenge yourself to expand. After all, there is more to life—and health—than just getting by. Neither the daily grind nor mindless amusement will ever make you truly happy. The reach is about taking the occasional leap.

For some of you, reaching might mean putting extra energy into disidentifying with a particular pathology (by quitting smoking or getting out of an addictive relationship). For you, going to twelve-step meetings or weekly therapy sessions would demonstrate your willingness to grow and develop. Or you might express your reach by practicing yoga or learning to dance or studying a foreign language. Anything that opens you up and makes you stronger and more self-aware.

The more you realize that life is about moving along your continuum of evolution, the easier it will be to prioritize your schedule in such a way that supports your growth and awakening. Keep taking your inventory, see where and how you could improve, and then take the steps to make it happen. Choose to expand. Strengthen your various intelligences and abilities in the areas of body, mind, and spirit. If you are doing well emotionally and are on a strong spiritual path, look to your health to see where you might upgrade. Or conversely, if you are fit and healthy but have no sense of spiritual purpose, pick up some books or open up a dialogue with someone who does. Push yourself to consider what isn't working (your sex life, friendships, or diet, to name a few areas); take responsibility where necessary, and then do what it takes to educate yourself so that you can be better.

Ask yourself these questions:

- **In which area(s) of my life do I most need to grow?**

- **What can I do that would support that growth?**

And then do it. If you feel well-balanced and nothing is screaming for your attention, go to the bookstore and feel yourself gravitate to the tomes that could teach you something. Pick out a lecture to attend in your community. Change up your mode of exercise. Try a new place of worship so that you can see how other people are inspired and then find some common ground.

I incorporate this reach sector into my schedule by reading a daily inspiration in one of the many books I have sitting at my bedside. I wake up, put on my glasses, and get inspired. And because I don't have a lot of time to read, the books that I choose are usually philosophical, self-help, or in some way informative. In this way, I am always learning something new so that my mind doesn't get lazy.

I also pray and meditate regularly, sometimes for only a few minutes and at other times for thirty minutes at a stretch. And throughout my adult life, I have sought out teachers, counselors, and therapists in various fields of healing; I like being "called out" on my stuff by someone objective who has my higher growth in mind. It's not always easy, and there are times when I just don't feel like working on myself, but for the most part I enjoy getting help and guidance.

Remember, too, that teachers come in many forms. Sometimes they appear through books, and sometimes they will pop up in a chance encounter. I've met a few sages in New York City taxis, believe it or not. Great spiritual teachers do not always wear robes and live in temples or lecture halls! As it is said, "When the student is ready, the teacher appears." So stay flexible, study, read, implement the new information, and keep thinking outside the norm. Spend your time with people you respect and who embody the qualities you want to have and learn from them. And remember that at times we grow out of relationships or situations. Let them go gently and with love.

Quantum wellness is clearly not a ho-hum endeavor; it requires a willingness to constantly evolve and upgrade. So think about who you are now and where you'd like to go. Sit down and map out your day with the big picture in mind. And then reach for it.

Try this:

1. **Make sure to attend to the four basic categories:**
   Regular: the everyday routines and obligations
   Relate: the extra attention that all relationships
   (work, partner, spouse, friend, child) require
   to be better and more fulfilling
   Rejuvenate: rest, receive, and restore

Reach: stretch past what is habitual and
comfortable

2. If you are an introvert, be sure that you get plenty of
downtime. You will feel most restored when you have quiet time
alone. If you are an extrovert, be sure to get the social interaction you need. That's what gives you your juice.

PART FOUR

Overcoming Obstacles

CHAPTER TEN

When You Are Faced with Crisis
Becoming Your Own Healer

I USED TO THINK THAT AS LONG AS I WAS A GOOD PERSON AND KEPT MY mind in a positive place, ate right, and did my spiritual work, I could steer clear of pain and suffering and enjoy a fruitful life. For the most part that's true. We reap positive results and consequences for the sound choices we make. But I have come to understand that sometimes things happen that are beyond our comprehension and that bad things do indeed happen to good people. Whether you call it karma from long ago, forgotten exchanges, or opportunities for growth, or even if you think of it as simply being caught up in the chaotic web of life, no matter how many wellness practices you have under your belt, you cannot be guaranteed that you will never have to deal with illness or other kinds of suffering. Your crisis may be physical, emotional, or spiritual; it may be related to your job, a relationship, or your health. No matter what the situation, you can become the healer who knows exactly what to do to get through it.

Things happen for reasons we can't know or understand: sometimes they make some sense while at other times we don't see the big picture or find meaning until after the crisis has passed. All kinds of people get sick or meet tragedy, no matter what kind of lives they lead. Even saints and sages encounter great trials, have health challenges, and eventually die. And just as these great souls struggle with and come through the darkness, so can we make our way through the dark times that may befall us.

I remember when my father lay dying in his hospital bed and he wondered aloud, "I must have done something really terrible to have to go through this." He hadn't done anything so terrible, of course; he was just trying to make sense of the cards he was dealt. But what he said really made me understand the anguish and confusion and chaos a person feels when trying to navigate the dark halls of a crisis. Nothing seems to make sense at times like these, and our best mechanisms for keeping our lives flowing along and under control may well be powerless against what's happening to us.

People get sick for many reasons, and it's often not clear what the cause really is: environmental factors—pesticides, herbicides, pollution, and food additives—may be harming our bodies without our realizing it. Stress, we know, sets off all kinds of internal responses and also depresses the immune system. Unhealed and unexpressed emotions fester and take their toll on our energy. Our genetic heritage sets us up for diseases. Nutritionless food that is processed and preserved with all sorts of chemicals may well be poisoning us. And there are viruses and bacteria floating around abundantly that can kick off any number of processes of inflammation or degeneration. No matter how well we defend ourselves against a potential malady—physical, mental, or spiritual—sometimes it just happens.

But we *can* do an awful lot to prevent disease or misfortune, including all the practices I've been discussing in this book. We can eat well and exercise and arm ourselves with information and tools and a force field of right attitude. We can surround ourselves with loving friends and a healthy environment. And we can stay informed and engaged in all things wellness oriented. If we make all these practices a part of our lives, then, if misfortune befalls us, we will be all the more ready to rise to meet our challenges in the smartest and most insightful way possible.

Should we become ill or have a setback on our wellness path, we have to reach beneath our familiar reserves and find resources of resilience and power that we may not know we have. It is as if we are called upon to act in ways that an authentic healer would (more on that soon), so that we not only coax forth the best possible result for the situation but also try to ensure that the experience, however difficult, is also a magnificent milestone along the path of our conscious evolution.

Magnificent milestone? What am I, crazy? Insincere? No, neither. I mean it. Being brought to our knees is often the catalyst for unimaginable breakthroughs. Think of Nelson Mandela and how he spent twenty-seven grueling years in prison before becoming the one who would successfully negotiate the dismantling of South African apartheid. And the Dalai Lama barely escaped with his life fleeing the oppression and threats aimed at him and his people; but with that loss he became a passionate and world-recognized leader of an even bigger aim: he is a guru not just of Tibetan Buddhism but also of the universal practices of kindness, forgiveness, and compassion. I'll bet you can think of a few examples of your own—times when you or someone you know has gone through some terrible time only to be brought into some deeper truth and strength. Again, we don't choose these experiences, but when they come, they come as teachers.

I do realize that this is tricky stuff.

People tend to get confused or angry when you broach the subject of the deeper meaning in illness or adversity. They think they are being blamed for their own illnesses. Nothing could be further from my intention. What I am talking about is tapping into the capability—not the culpability—of the Healer within each and every one of us. This Healer with a capital H is the part of you who can strike the mystical balance between accepting what is and taking the proactive steps whispered to you by your highest intuition. The Healer witnesses the truth of what is and then divines the right solution. She takes matters into her own hands.

Just recently I sat down with a distant cousin of mine who told me the story of how her daughter Margie had accidently rolled her car over her little three-year-old son, killing him instantly. I sat stunned and transfixed as my cousin recounted the saddest details of the ordeal her daughter went through upon realizing what she had done. In the months following the death of her child, Margie's guilt and grief voraciously ate away at her faith in God and took a heavy toll on her health and marriage. Here was a woman who was good and kind and had lived her life in a way that hurt no one. And yet something so unspeakably horrible and random happened and everything was suddenly turned upside down. A spiritual crisis had come upon her, to say the least. Margie barely ate or slept, and for long stretches of time she stayed curled up in a ball, engulfed by her sorrow. Margie wanted to die and wished that her body would just cease to function.

But the minister of her church visited her daily, bringing her words of consolation and a promise that there was something more than met the eye, that healing was possible. Gradually he helped Margie accept and grieve over what happened. He told her that God would assuage her guilt and receive her rage.

So Margie kept wailing and screaming and rocking and wimpering, giving to her God what the minister said He would take. And ever so slowly, Margie began to experience moments—and then stretches of moments—of peace. The minister assured her that she would one day come to realize that God did not find her guilty but rather saw her innocence. And in that vein, she could perhaps forgive herself. It was the slightest ray of light, but light it was.

After a few months, Margie joined an online support group for parents who had gone through similar situations. At first she just signed on, but slowly she began to participate in the conversation. She then found that by taking long walks she could connect with the spirit of her son. She would just walk and talk with what felt like his spirit and the deep grief began to lift. She found herself wanting to reach out to a few of the group's newcomers, who had more recently experienced a tragedy, and thus began to feel, as she said, "almost useful."

Eventually Margie agreed to go to counseling with her husband, and they both started keeping a journal of what was happening within and around them. She returned to her old job and added some volunteer work to keep her nights and weekends busy.

All this happened gradually and incrementally, small breakthroughs occurring spontaneously throughout the process.

Margie feels that this awful loss brought her into a relationship with God, and that the lessons the little boy had come to teach her were about forgiveness, healing, and compassion. Everyone I've met who has lost a small child says the same thing: there is no other experience that compares—not losing a spouse or a parent or personally suffering a severe accident, nothing. Margie agrees, and although obviously she would give the world to have her son back, she is convinced that the horrible experience and the depths to which it brought her taught her lessons she could not have learned in any other way.

Margie says she has come to understand in a visceral, lived way that healing comes from acceptance, expression of truth, compassion, and service. She now gives talks all around the country inspiring people to grow through their crises and become the healers they are capable of being.

Margie's experience was extreme, yes. It was so unfair, so tragic. But I tell it because even after that great tragedy, she was able to go through the alchemical process of turning darkness into something beautiful and light. Margie became a healer, not by choice but by rising—slowly and authentically—to the occasion that presented itself. As a footnote, Margie and her husband had another child, and they are thriving as a family. And her son, Margie says, remains the angel guiding her path.

So how do we cope with the dual realities of accepting what is and becoming proactive in a way that calls forth a miracle? That's the key question. We do it by extracting the vital energy from both surrender and focused action.

The following is a guide that can help you through a crisis, or even just through the inevitable day-to-day challenges that can otherwise nip at our heels and ultimately deplete us.

Accept What Is

The first step is to figure out how to stay present to whatever is arising in the moment. When we do this, we stop lying to ourselves or hoping for something to be different and instead take in the facts of the situation, however grave, and feel all the feelings that come up. Rather than becoming fogged in by denial, we choose to remain rooted in truth—even when that truth is looking very ugly.

Of course this may be simply impossible for you, especially when a crisis first hits. You may have to sink for a while, like Margie did. But it sure can help to keep trying to pull your attention back to the present moment, if you can.

This means that if you are asked how you are doing after being diagnosed with a serious ailment, for instance, you do not force a stiff upper lip and say "Fine." You speak the truth of what you are feeling (at least to yourself if not out loud or to others you don't feel safe with) or perhaps just acknowledge that you are not ready to talk about it. That's okay, too. But when we try to fake being positive, we deny our truth. When we don't admit to feelings—of anger or despair or fear—we can't respond to the moment in a clear way because we are too busy suppressing what's uncomfortable.

Suppressing emotions is one of those survival mechanisms; we often don't even know we're doing it. But we can learn to interrupt that unconscious pattern by pausing and listening to our inner selves with the intention of allowing anything and everything to become conscious. Emotions remain dangerous when they are held underground, and they lose their destructive power when they are brought to consciousness. If you doubt this, I urge you to try feeling those scary feelings, starting with a situation that's relatively uncomplicated.

As you become attuned to what is happening in the moment, bearing witness to the part of you that is afraid or full of anguish, a gust of intuition will blow through you. Your presence will call forth new responses from within, thus increasing your healing aptitude. Keep all your senses open to new information. You will hear the name of the perfect person to call, which specialist to trust, and what to do. It will flash through your mind as a sudden memory or pop up in a conversation or in an article you glance at in the checkout line. Pay attention. These are missives from the Healer within, who takes charge in crises. If you are emotionally present and committed to tapping into your highest and deepest awareness, you will hear the voice of Spirit within you, guiding you to the next right step. That's just the way we work. We are always evolving, always discovering how vastly intelligent life is. As you find your way toward the right path for a physical turnaround, you will also be touched by the grace of Spirit, which is always purifying and lifting your energy.

When we try to keep fear at bay because we think it would be better to "let it go" or "be brave," we actually feed the energy of the very thing that stands in the way of our progress. Suppressing difficult feelings is hard work.

It's time to open, to go deep. Every time you are tempted to shut down, breathe deeply and listen. Find compassion for the parts of you that are suffering. Facing the suffering is what will alleviate the fear, not turning away from it. In fact, when you do this, when you face your fear, you discover that there is nothing *to* fear, because the worst is happening and you are actually okay.

You might not want to feel the full extent of your sadness or the depth of the rage that lurks beneath that veil of control, but I urge you to turn toward the feelings anyway. Breathe into them. Express them in a way that feels comfortable and safe. Try it. They will soon begin to lose their charge.

I have a friend named Chelsea who was recently diagnosed with breast cancer. She was terrified, to say the least, and set about doing everything an educated woman would do in order to get the best possible treatment. She found a top-notch surgeon and oncologist, immediately cleaned up her diet, started working with a meditation counselor, and practiced doing positive affirmations. But when I asked her what was going on inside her emotionally, I noticed that she tightened her jaw a bit when she said that she was doing the best that she could. When I see someone's jaw clench, I think of anger, because that is one of the ways the body holds it. So I asked her, "Are you angry about this?" She said that she didn't have time for anger, that it served no purpose and that she only wanted to stay in a "good" place. When I explained to her that a "good" place was an honest place, she relented and began to open up.

Chelsea had a lot of responsibilities: Her husband was a perfectionist and somewhat demanding, her children were in constant need of attention, and her friends all looked to her to be the voice of reason and wisdom. She was always there for her parents and siblings, and her kids' school had come to count on her for her ability to organize various functions. The more she gave voice to these things, the more angry she felt at how much of herself she was always giving away. It wasn't that she was creating *more* anger by allowing it to surface, she was just finally getting in touch with the anger she already felt. And then, by becoming aware of it, she was able to attend to some things that had been out of balance for a long, long time.

She decided to hand over the duties at the school to someone else, stood up to her husband when he started in on his faultfinding, and gently let her family and friends know that she was going to kick back for a while from her regular role of "the all-knowing, all-helping one."

She didn't dump on anyone or become a so-called rager, she just took some thoughtful steps to lighten her load and focus a little more on herself. And by becoming authentic, she was led to a more meaningful place as she faced her cancer and her healing.

Chelsea says she felt "fierce" when she tapped into her truth, as if this strength to say no had just been waiting for release. She says she felt freer and lighter. The truth of her cancer didn't change, at least not right away, but she began to operate at a more authentic level, a higher level.

That's what happens when we simply listen to what's going on inside us and honor it responsibly. The way is illuminated.

It is our highest calling to look directly at the darkness within us and bring it to light. We won't necessarily make instant peace with it, no. But if we recognize and observe the darkness and meet it with acceptance, we become more fully integrated and at peace with ourselves. We position ourselves for the quantum shift.

Guiding Yourself Out of Panic

If you find yourself with a serious diagnosis or other bad news, just try to stay present with whatever you are feeling. That's the first step. Keep asking yourself, "What am I feeling now? What is arising in me now?" and then meet those feelings and thoughts with a nod. "Okay,

I see. I breathe into that. I allow that to be so." That kind of radical acceptance transmutes negativity, and you find yourself feeling okay no matter what.

Here are four steps that can help you through panic.

1. **Focus on your breath.** Just take several slow, deep, easy breaths. As you inhale, wherever there is tightness imagine the breath just moving into and relaxing the area of stress. Once you've taken the breath as far as you can, hold it for just one more moment before exhaling audibly through your mouth. At the place of transition between inhaling and exhaling, sense yourself tapping into a golden light of healing. Bring that light into your breath as you exhale fully, visualizing the light being spread throughout your body and into your challenging circumstance. Just see the light being poured into all the dark recesses of fear and anxiety. Repeat the inhale, pausing at the end to tap into and gather more light, and then exhale again. Do this until you feel calm.

2. **Explore all the possibilities.** Allow yourself to think of the best and worst possible outcomes. Say you have a diagnosis of a potentially fatal disease. Ask yourself, "What is the worst thing that can happen?" Here is what the progression of thought might sound like: *"The worst thing that could happen is that I will die a slow and agonizing death. And lose all my money along the way. My children will be frightened and I will become a burden to those I love."* It doesn't get any worse than that, so now your energy is freed up for more proactive uses. Here might be the next phase of the thought process: *"Well, the truth is that everybody dies. At some point, I will be facing my death, so I might as well look into the possibility. I know only this external world, but there is a whole other level—probably many levels—of reality that is yet to be explored. That exploration may actu-*

ally be a wonderful experience. If pain is involved, I can take the medication. And as much as I don't want to lose my material possessions, if that is the lesson I am meant to learn—that money comes and goes, or that you can't hold on to anything, or that every attachment is meant to be confronted—then I will rise to that challenge. And as for my children, I wish they didn't have to experience any of this, but we are all born with our cross to bear. I have to believe that this is all part of some great plan that will enrich my family and me. My children will learn compassion from this; and they will be deepened by what they witness. I hate being a burden, but perhaps the lesson for me is that I can learn how to receive when otherwise I felt uncomfortable doing so."

Allow your mind to take you right into the very worst that it can be, and then find the light. Make peace with whatever life throws at you. By doing this, you are not prolonging your suffering by worrying; you are going straight into your fears and dealing with them. Most of the time, things will never even remotely approach what you feared they might, but by being prepared for anything and everything, you can more easily move through the fear and into healing.

On the flip side, be sure to explore the possibility that everything will turn out really well. People get misdiagnosed all the time. I have a friend who was told by his doctor that he had a fatal disease and had only six months left to live. He was devastated. So he thought about how he wanted to live out the rest of his life, and he moved to Rome to live it up. Six months passed, and then a year. He went to a doctor over there and found out that he didn't have the disease at all; his scans had somehow been read incorrectly and he was completely fine.

There are spontaneous healings that can't be explained, new treatments offered, and alternative methods from cultures other than ours that are extremely effective. You just don't know what kind of miracle could unfold in your case, but once you start exploring the possibilities, you might realize that you also have a chance at experiencing one.

3. Ask Spirit to come into the situation and take over. Saying a prayer will help you to remember that you are not in this alone, that in fact there is a benevolent force that is always available to us when we call on it. The prayer might sound something like this: *"Dear Spirit, I ask that you make your presence known here and now, for I am very frightened and don't know what to do or how to handle things. Please infuse my being with your light, surround me with your love, that I may be lifted up and carried by your grace. Whisper into my thinking the inspirations that will help me through this. Help me to be clear and calm. Embolden my heart with the courage to stay present and connected, for I know that in that presence lies my healing. I ask you to guide me—and everyone involved in this situation— every step of the way. Lift my spirit into a higher vibration that I might grow from this experience and become my greatest potential. Let there be a miracle. I am open and willing to have a miracle occur. Let the healer within me rise and take charge. I thank you in advance as I know that it is already so."*

The more you can sincerely reach out and ask for help—not only from Spirit but also in spiritual fellowship from friends or a support system—the more you will relax knowing that, on a very real level, everything is being taken care of. Go to places where you feel most in touch with your spiritual nature. Sit in a church or temple; walk through a meadow or wade into the gentle current of a river. Hang out with your animal companions. Visit a guru or spiritual teacher whom you respect. Soak up all the positive energy you can find and let it carry you through this difficult time.

4. Resolve to make a plan. Decide to do whatever is necessary to promote your healing. Research and write down all the steps you might take. Find out who the experts are in your area of need, and read everything they have written on the subject. Scour the Internet for natural and alternative solutions so that your approach is an integrated one. Talk to people who have gone through what you are encountering and note what worked for them; ask for their recommendations on books, workshops, or classes. At this point, write down your plan. That will allow your mind to move on to other important aspects of your recovery without having to worry that you will forget something. Make a list of everything you want to do or check out, and cross things off the list as you accomplish them. This will keep you engaged in your own therapeutic process, which will help you to remain feeling like a powerful actor rather than a passive victim.

You may have noticed that the first letters of these four steps spell out the word *fear*. It's a good mnemonic: focus (on your breath), explore (the possibilities—both positive and negative), ask (for guidance from Spirit), and resolve (to make a plan).

Be Proactive

As much as it is vital to "be with what is" when dealing with any kind of critical predicament, it is equally important to be proactive, to find your way *through* the situation at hand and not just become a victim of circumstance. Being proactive obviously means getting second or third opinions, making yourself an expert on the condition you find yourself in, and changing your lifestyle or health regimen in all the relevant ways. But the real essence of being proactive is that you stay engaged and committed to keeping your energy flowing, thus stoking the fire of the healing response.

Here are a few more tips for keeping your energy moving in a positive direction:

1. Be open to the prospect of healing. It's easy to feel doomed and distressed when we get bad news, and that's okay. As you experience everything that comes up, remind yourself that there is every possibility that things can turn out very well; they very often do.

People heal from terrible circumstances all the time, in ways both conventional and surprising. Some will say it was an herb or a diet that did the trick; others will tell you they found a great doctor. Almost all of them will tell you they "just had a feeling" that some sort of miracle was brewing. You don't have to be fully convinced that one method or the other will work for you, and you don't have to maintain a positive attitude at all times. But you must be willing to believe that all things *are* possible, including your miraculous (or gentle, or rapid, or easy) recovery. Again, sometimes healing happens on the physical plane, while other times it is more of a spiritual awakening. Your soul will guide you if you remain receptive to the enlightenment that calls you. Say to yourself at least once an hour, "I am open to healing. I am willing to experience a miracle."

2. Process your grievances. It's really important to clear out all the old resentments, guilty feelings, and unresolved issues, as these are the psychic blockages that catch at the healing energy that wants to flow through you. Think about who you have not forgiven and process your anger or hurt in a responsible way. Write a scathing letter that you don't send; scream into the sky where no one can hear you. Picture the person(s) in front of you and give them a piece of your mind. And then ask Spirit to assist you in seeing them for the wounded people they are, that you may finally know they did only the best they could with what they had. If you can't imagine forgiving the person, picture communicating with his soul and letting him know that your intention is to move forward unencumbered by ill will.

And on the other hand, where you feel guilty, make amends and clean up whatever mess you might have created with another person. Now is the time to be vulnerable and say you are sorry. It's not easy to face someone you know you have hurt, but having done so, you will feel lighter and freer to accept good things happening to you. Often, we unconsciously punish ourselves because we consider ourselves "bad," feeling we did something awful and deserve to be penalized. When you make amends, the person on the receiving end can finally move on also, and you will most likely feel the goodwill coming back to you. Whatever grievances you don't feel safe or comfortable airing out directly with the person, journal them through as if you are speaking directly to them. Clear the slate and make room for fresh energy.

3. Make a list of everything that might add to the momentum of healing, and then tick off each suggestion as you do it. When we are caught up in the chaos of dealing with a serious diagnosis, we can easily forget the simplest things that could buoy us. So eat, watch a funny movie, call your best friend, snuggle with your dog. These simple joys will lift your energy and remind you why life is worth living. Do things that nourish you: get a massage, take a salt bath, move your body to get your circulation going, breathe lots of fresh air. All these activities send a signal to the universe (and to your unconscious) that you are opening up rather than closing down. Besides, doing joyful things actually calls forth our optimism. Every time a smile breaks across your face, the entire energy of your body lifts. You don't have to force yourself to be positive, just do things that will authentically make you happy. As Dr. Bernie Siegel says in his book *Peace, Love, and Healing*, there really is a "physiology of optimism . . . and joy." He says that "anything that offers hope has the potential to heal."

Read inspiring books, let a priest or monk or rabbi bless you, chant in the woods with a shaman who channels healing. Whatever feels good and joyous and hopeful, do it, not out of desperation but out of a willingness to participate on every level of your healing.

4. Make suggestions to your body about ways it could heal. You can contribute to your own healing process by focusing the workings of your body in certain ways. You can picture your heart slowing down and beating regularly; you can imagine a tumor dissolving and un-raveling itself from an organ; you can ask your lungs to relax and open up; you can suggest that your blood circulate more freely and vibrantly. You can ask your emotional state to deliver its communiqué and then release you from anxiety or depression. Sometimes the body (and mind) just needs a little direction, and since they are so intricately con-nected, we really can shift our inner workings by simply focusing on balance and flow. I'm not saying you can just picture your health and be cured, but you *can* repattern the energy that is moving throughout your emotional and physical body by tuning in to it and subtly sug-gesting a shift.

When you make these suggestions, do so without desperation or an attachment to seeing results. It is more a matter of leaning into the condition and then unkinking the energy where it is stuck or knotted. Approach this work from a loving space, accepting what is going on but trusting that the divine Healer works not only through doctors and medicines, but through you and for you.

5. Keep a body-mind-spirit journal. Whenever you notice your mind whirling in emotional chaos, take out your journal and write fast and furiously. Don't think about it; don't try to sound poetic or smart. Just write straight from the heart with the intention of becoming more attuned to your Truth. Give every part of you a chance to express itself. Truths will just pop out on the paper. You will uncover issues or areas that need to be addressed or tended to. A memory will come up that you can finally cry over—and then let go of. You might realize that you are angrier than you ever cared to admit—and can now take steps to repair. And you might very well discover a depth of feeling that you didn't know you had because thoughts and emotions will pour out of you when given a safe place to express.

6. Take a few minutes a day to reflect on whom and what you love and appreciate. Healing requires a delicate balance of being real with what's happening and keeping the fire of motivation stoked. Focus on the good things you have enjoyed thus far—warm friendships, a cozy home, even a favorite meal. This will enhance the positive force field of energy that swirls around and throughout you.

7. Do something for someone else. You'll recall from our Eight Pillars discussion of service that reaching outside yourself will take your focus off your fear. Help your nephew tie his shoe, tell a friend why you think he is wonderful, feed the parking meter or pay a bridge toll for someone you don't even know; all these things will make you feel good about yourself. You will feel alive and useful, and you will feel good karma coming your way. By being the Healer for someone else, you will realize the power you have and can begin to use it on yourself.

By striking a balance between *being with what is* and *staying proactive*, you will find yourself taking a quantum leap toward a new level of wellness. You can use these tools with any crisis or challenging situation: if you are betrayed by a loved one, or lose your job, or are struggling with some wicked inner demons, keep letting go while pushing through all at the same time. Go within even as you reach out. These hard times are the challenges that inspire us to listen and show up in ways we never did before. Life is coaxing us to grow into and realize our full potential as spiritual human beings, so assume this crisis is here to deliver you somehow. As much as you can, keep opening your heart and remain willing to shift into a higher gear.

Surely we would prefer to have life neatly organized around black-and-white truths: if we do all the right things, life will turn out just the way we want it to. The flaw in this thinking, of course, is the assumption that we are in total control of our lives. We are not. We are indeed powerful creators of our own destiny, but we are not the sole creators. We work in tandem with Spirit as we navigate the maze of our past karma (the law of cause and effect of each action ever done), the inevitable stickiness of a world with countless egos criss-crossing one another's paths, and the unknowable web of chaos that is inherent in a rapidly unfolding universe. We are being shaped into richer and more soulful human beings. Sometimes this process of evolution happens through gentle recognition of a truth revealed, while at other times revelations are more hard-won.

If things seem as if they are falling apart for you, assume grace and wisdom are on the way, and keep looking for what the experience is trying to teach you. It *will* be revealed.

Try this:

Anytime you find yourself gripped with fear, remember:

F—Focus on your breathing.
E—Explore all the possibilities and make peace with them.
A—Ask for spiritual assistance.
R—Resolve to take all the pertinent steps.

When you find yourself in the maze of a crisis, whether the challenge is illness, injury, a work conflict, or relationship fallout:

1. Be open to the prospect of healing.
2. Process your grievances.
3. Make a list of everything you can do that will add to the momentum of healing.
4. Make suggestions to your body on how it can heal.
5. Keep a journal.
6. Reflect on whom and what you love and appreciate.
7. Do something for someone else.

CHAPTER ELEVEN

More Detours on the Wellness Path
Breaking Bad Habits

ANOTHER OBSTACLE TO WELLNESS THAT OFTEN FLIES UNDER THE RADAR is addiction and dependency. There are, of course, the obvious addictions like alcohol and cigarettes and cocaine. But we humans are prone to addiction in many forms: we get addicted to relationship drama, to gambling or shopping or sex or checking e-mail or politics or eating or even to taking care of other people. Whatever it is we do habitually to keep us numbed or distracted from deeper emotional truths can be considered an addiction. Even those of us who consider ourselves fairly far along on a wellness path can be caught up in unhealthy dependencies and thus blocked from the full experience of wellness. We will never experience the quantum breakthroughs until we break these destructive habits and discover the purpose they have been serving for us.

Addictions often start off as fun or stress-relieving distractions—drinking with your buddies in the spirit of camaraderie or to unwind, shopping online to reward yourself for a stressful day or week at work, or pigging out on a Saturday night alone, for example—but they can easily escalate into all-consuming urges that provide diminishing returns in terms of relief while piling on the shame. No matter what habit has a hold on you, if it is adversely impacting your work life and relationships, you need help and you would be wise to get it. If you are drinking or using drugs or doing anything else so much that you feel sick or miss work or your loved ones are complaining, that is enough of an indication that addiction is present and in need of attention. Universally, recovering addicts will say that what helps them overcome is group support or counseling (or both). It can't hurt to try it, and if you're resistant, that's another indication that you have a problem that needs addressing. Our culture so values the "pull yourself up by your own bootstraps" ethic, but there is nothing shameful about having an addiction. Look at it, instead, as a doorway into your awakening.

Most sober addicts will tell you that their addiction helped them to grow spiritually, but only once they got help.

Perhaps you don't think of yourself as an addict. And perhaps you are not. But you might want to read through the following section and see if you recognize yourself at all. You might be surprised. As I mentioned, addictions can take many forms. In fact I sometimes prefer the term *negative habituations*, because it covers a broader field of compulsive and destructive thoughts and behaviors.

We know we have an addiction when we find ourselves unhealthfully preoccupied by a substance, behavior, or person in such a way that our relationships, work, and health begin to suffer. You know you are addicted when your life revolves around something that severely diminishes your energy and yet you can't (or won't) stop it. Addictions have the effect of numbing us out and distancing us from something painful. You'll find yourself denying that you have a problem ("It's just shopping! I don't *have* to do it" or "I am totally in control; I simply choose to get stoned every night after work" or "I just like having a lot of sex; I'm not an addict just because I've had a lot of lovers lately") even as the quality of your life gets worse with each passing week or year. Whatever your fatal attraction, at best it keeps you in a holding pattern and away from thriving in all your power, and at worst it puts you in a fast-moving downward spiral, in which you can lose your job, your home, your family.

Some people are lucky and slowly wake up to the fact that things have to change if they want to survive; but there are many others who have to be brought to their knees. They have to bottom out before waking up—by losing a job or marriage, by getting arrested and publicly humiliated, by having their bodies fail them because they can no longer tolerate the abuse. As awful as it sounds, this bottoming out, or what Saint John of the Cross first called the dark night of the soul, is often a doorway to healing.

When we are desperate and afraid—that's when we finally become willing to take a look under the hood and fix what's broken.

Paradoxically, we often become addicted—whether it be to alcohol, sugary foods, video games, cigarettes, or lovers—in order to transcend a lower state of being. We are trying to resolve a spiritual crisis by doing something that makes us feel good, to ease the uncomfortable feelings that threaten to consume us. Indeed, if we drink enough or eat enough or gamble enough, we will experience a temporary blotting out of the voices of self-loathing that are nipping at the edge of our awareness. It is certainly understandable to want to escape, to reach for something that will give us a few minutes or hours of relative peace and transcendence. But those dark voices—the ones that tell us we are not good enough in one way or another—will never lose their charge when pushed down and away; they just fester and gather steam until they can make their way to the surface again. And they only tend to get louder and more insistent.

These voices—even though they may have originated from a parent or some other early influence—are now part of us; they are intricately and inextricably woven throughout our psyche. They influence our every thought, behavior, and relationship whether we are conscious of it or not. But these dark sentiments cannot forever be shoved down by our addictive behaviors; eventually we have to deal with them squarely, soberly, and lovingly. Only by listening and applying the antidote of emotional presence can the negative charge dissipate in a real and lasting way.

The poetic and twisted irony of addictive behaviors is that they ultimately sabotage the very state of being we are striving for—peace and transcendence—because they are false gods, idols if you will, unable to give us anything but fleeting distraction. And we become enslaved to them. We allow them to dictate our lives; we revolve around them and make them our top priority, sacrificing everything to protect our access to them. Although we look to them to save us, they end up sucking the life right out of us.

Indulging an addiction or negative habituation is an understandable grab at having a better experience of life, but it never works for long. It can't, because we are meant to come to know the true Spirit, the love within and all around us—our connectedness with Spirit and with each other. False gods will always be exposed for what they are—hollow promises of deliverance.

You may or may not be dealing with addiction at this time in your life, but most of us do indeed pass through periods of obsession or compulsion in one way or another. These fixations, whether we are wrestling with them directly or living with someone who is, hold us back from experiencing our full potential for all-around wellness.

When we are consumed by the cycle of addiction, pursuing wellness through good eating practices, healthy relating, and serving a higher purpose in the world can't possibly stay on the front burner. How can you focus on upping the ante of your physical capabilities when all you can think about is your next dose or the cake you'll reward yourself with when you've worked out? How can you make your mark in the world when your energy is otherwise occupied with a relationship drama that goes round and round? If you want to move forward in any sort of substantial way, you have to address your demons. The good news is, though, that like everything, this struggle serves a great purpose in that it gets you to look more deeply at what is working and what is not so that you can make choices that support your evolution.

In this big-picture perspective, addiction can have a useful role on our wellness continuum. If it doesn't kill us first (and I say this so that you feel the full brunt of how serious addiction can be), it can often be a catalyst for growth, because it is so pressing a problem that we have to dig very deep inside to figure out how to stop it. We have to come to terms with old memories or beliefs and at last clear away the destructive energy holding it in place. We have to upgrade the way we eat, rest, and commune; and we have to give birth to a fresher, purer version of ourselves.

The soul will always seek to expand and deepen; that is its nature. Our addictions, if we let them, will teach us what we need to know about surrender, presence, diligence, and humility—the very qualities that will round us out and illumine us as human beings.

I don't presume to be able to break your addictions through this book. You may well need to get professional help or seek out local resources such as Alcoholics Anonymous. But I would like to outline a few steps that are helpful in addressing and healing an addiction, as they are a little different from the ones you would use with an illness or other tragedy. A little different, but not entirely. (Please note that these are *not* intended to replace the twelve-step process of AA; in fact, some of them are akin to them. They are meant to be an adjunct to whatever path you choose to take.)

1. Recognize that you have a problem. Half the battle in dealing with addiction lies in simply admitting that you have a problem that has gotten out of hand. If you get uncomfortable and out of sorts when you are unable to satisfy a craving, you might want to ask yourself if you have an addiction or unhealthy compulsion. I have a friend, Joe, who could not relax unless he had his scotch and soda at the end of the day. If for some reason he got to a restaurant or friend's home and his drink wasn't handy, Joe would get very agitated and wouldn't be able to focus on even the simplest conversation. After about fifteen minutes, he would start looking angry and panicked and then make an excuse to leave. But if he had a few drinks, he was able to relax and be his regular gregarious self.

When Joe's doctor told him that he had to stop drinking because his liver was enlarged and toxic, he scoffed at the idea and kept right on going. He ended up losing his job after coming to work late too many times, but he blamed the boss for being "uptight." When he was stopped for drunk driving and issued a DUI for the second time, Joe blamed the California police for being overly vigilant and not chasing after "real" criminals. Finally, when his beloved wife packed her bags and told him she had had enough, Joe decided he had a problem with his drinking and sought help.

Once you can see the destructive effects of your addiction, you can begin to make an honest attempt at turning things around. If someone just pushes you into rehab without your being on board, recovery doesn't stand much of a chance. *You* have to see that your addiction is causing you to suffer. You won't change until you come out of denial.

When Joe admitted that he had a problem, all sorts of resources began to open up for him. His cousin called to share with him his own experience with alcoholism and offered to take him to some twelve-step meetings. His wife decided to give him another chance if he agreed to check himself into rehab within the week, and a group of his closest friends stepped in to tell him how much they had worried about him, but how they would help him through this period of recovery if he would remain open and honest about his addiction.

Although this was a humiliating experience for him at first, Joe began to realize that he was deeply loved and had a lot to lose if he didn't work on himself. So he took the offers of help and guidance and basked in the respect that his peers reflected back to him. It is always excruciatingly difficult to admit that we have a problem and have been going about things in the wrong way, but once we do, we can stop trying to hold everything together by ourselves and start relying on a support system (such as friends, family, a treatment center, a fellowship program), all of which, we will discover, is infinitely more dependable than the substance or behavior we were addicted to.

If you suspect you are an addict in some way, ask yourself if you are truly free to give it up, and then stop. Be honest with yourself. Check yourself out: Do you feel a nearly uncontrollable urge to pick up the habit again? Do you find yourself making excuses? Does your well-being seem dependent on having access to your habit, and then is it quickly dashed when the habit doesn't seem to make things better, but worse? If you feel worn down by the cycle of longing, acting out, and then shame, just try admitting to yourself that you have a problem. As difficult as it is to reach this point, consider that perhaps the negative fallout that you have suffered has been a necessary part of your path to wellness. It reduced you to a humble state, thereby readying you for a conversion experience. This honest assessment really is the foundation for spiritual awakening.

2. Be willing to do things differently. Most people who suffer with addiction don't know that things can be any other way than they are. They feel trapped by their compulsions and sense that their fate is locked into some downward spiral that can't be stopped. And the truth is, unless we do something different, the same scenario will indeed play out over and over again. Before any change can be made though, there has to be willingness. You have to at least be open to the *idea* that you could live another way, that you might one day have different instincts, healthier cravings, and better ways of coping. You will need help, of course, in getting to the place where you can experience release from the habit, but your free will must be engaged. You are absolutely free to choose difficulty and chaos; you can keep doing what you are doing and progress along the dark path of addiction until you hit bottom so hard that you wake up. Or you could, like Joe, say to yourself, *Okay; I have a problem. I don't know how to fix it yet; but I am willing to consider that there may be another way of doing things. My intention is to heal and overcome this glitch on my path; I no longer want to be enslaved to this negative habituation that I've engaged in. I am open to seeing things differently and to act in ways that empower me to become a healthier person.*

Joe saw that he had a choice. He didn't immediately know how to change the course of his life, but he was willing to consider that the miracle of healing was available to him if he cooperated. He knew he didn't have all the answers (or any of the answers for that matter!), but he was willing to remain open to the healthy guidance that came his way.

There is an almost magical element that is unleashed when you open the door and invite in help. Once we say, "Okay, I'm ready to grow—give me your best shot," all kinds of synchronicities and benevolent help will come flooding in through this opening. You begin to realize that the only thing that was blocking your good was you. And when you step aside, it's as if the whole universe comes around to support you. You will sense in the air an almost mystical quality that feels like you have aligned yourself with the force of growth and good and you will most likely feel a gentle optimism take over as you give up trying to hold everything together.

You don't have to *do* anything at this point, just remain open and willing to do things differently.

Sometimes you only have to sit with this step for a little while before you are ready to move forward, but with most people it takes weeks or months of just hovering in the state of "willingness" before your energy shifts from "I know what is best and I'll be damned if I'm going to change" to "Maybe I don't know what is best, so I'll just hold to the intention of becoming healthy and I'll do whatever it takes to support that intention." Trust that you are well on your way.

3. Connect with Spirit. However you choose to picture Spirit, it is a simple truth that we all spring from the same universal life force that breathes through us and enlivens us, and we can tap into it anytime we want to by getting quiet and sensing its mystery. We all have an inborn intelligence that pushes us toward our highest good. When you connect with this force, with Spirit, you align with the creative life force.

Call this energy what you will—Jesus, Buddha, Allah, Divine Mother, or whatever feels right to you. Atheists may simply refer to the loving, unifying power we experience within ourselves and with each other. The point is, we all have access to it every moment of every day. Call out to it and eventually, you will begin to feel free of even religious confines and touch on your own light, feeling the seed of Spirit within you.

If you are not sure that Spirit is there for you, try out a simple prayer and see how it feels. Just say "Spirit, please help me." And then rest in knowing that you reached out. You will most likely feel a sense of calm and hopefulness, as if something inside you knows that you did the right thing. Spiritual connection takes practice; to just go on faith alone can leave you feeling empty and doubtful. It is quite possible that right now you feel let down by Spirit, that if Spirit had been there for you, things wouldn't have gotten as out of hand as they are. Or the world wouldn't be in the state that it's in. But we have to remember that much of where the world is today is the result of human misbehavior. We have free will, and if we don't rise to a higher evolution of ourselves, life will simply reflect our poor choices.

If we have been victimized and wounded in our lives (and these are the forces that often give us reason to act out with our addictions in the first place), we certainly have the right to feel angry or sad or afraid. But we don't have to continually make decisions that will further our misery; we can step out and risk trusting again. We can reach out to the kindness and wisdom of new friends or counselors with the aim of restoring our connection to the Source, which is love. In reaching out, we will begin to gravitate toward those who have a more solid sense of spiritual connection. That love and trust will sink in. We will become ever more aware that there is indeed a "power greater than ourselves" that we can look to for support. Let your prayers get more detailed; one might sound like this: *Dear Spirit, my life has become so confusing and chaotic. I don't know what to do anymore, but I am willing to be guided and inspired. May my thoughts become more serene. May my actions and communications become more stable and loving. May my heart remain open as I find my way into a sober and joyful life. Thank you. Amen.* Your life will begin to change. It will be as if some powerful force is backing your every effort to move toward health; you will gather strength, clarity, and momentum as you move toward your next step.

4. **Stay in the moment.** For any addict, there is a moment right before you use that feels unbearable. It is usually some form of anxiety

that is accompanied by an extremely unpleasant feeling. You may feel worried or angry or hopeless; you may have just had a difficult conversation or your memory has taken you back to a time that deeply injured you. As these thoughts and emotions well up, the natural instinct is to blot them out; you want to make it all go away and stop the uncomfortable feeling. So here is the turning point. If you are tempted to flee, cover up, or numb out, instead breathe into the very thing that feels threatening. Just breathe into it and *stay with it*. When I say stay, I mean let whatever wants to arise, arise. Allow yourself the feelings, explore the memory, or observe the chatter that's going on in your brain without trying to change the subject. Instead of turning away, turn into it and allow it to be there in all its ugly glory. This may sound antithetical to the positive thinking we are all encouraged to do these days, but I don't believe you can ever really get to that optimistic state until all the other parts of you have made their peace.

If we want to transform our suffering rather than eternally trying to outrun it (which we can't), we have to be with it mindfully. We have to look and listen to all the dark parts of ourselves with a compassionate ear. By looking squarely at our wounds and letting ourselves feel everything that comes along with them, with the intent of using them for our eventual transformation, we gain compassion for ourselves, and this ends up opening our heart and making us more available to love. This process makes our human journey rich and worthwhile.

Pain will not go away on its own; it needs to be tended to. When we lovingly stay in the moment, we salve our wounds. We transform the suffering into compassion so that we don't keep playing out the same old dark drama.

Going back to my friend Joe, the urge to drink would sneak up on him like a slow itch until it became a nearly violent desire. Once he knew he was an addict and became committed to being sober, he would say his prayers in these agonizing moments, visualizing an army of angels gathering around to support him as he settled into the boiling rage that he had always feared would consume him. Joe had had a very difficult childhood and his pain was easily triggered when anyone showed him even the slightest bit of disapproval. But he learned to stay with the uncomfortable feelings, breathing into them as he screamed at the top of his lungs (this only in a safe environment, of course) and eventually dissolved into tears. He began to notice that these spells became less frequent and had less of a charge to them. He learned that he could get through them and even came to see them as turning points in his spiritual evolution.

Slowly, Joe began to develop a great compassion for the child he was who had to deal with such traumatic abuse; it's not that he wallowed in self-pity but rather grew in self-esteem as he saw how far he had come. The childhood wound that resulted in his adult addiction was, in this way, his foundation for growth; it was his sacred soft spot. His despair ultimately brought him humility and empathy when he addressed it consciously, thus he became a healer to himself and, later, to others.

The next time you feel tempted to use your drug of choice, pause for a moment, connect to Spirit, and let yourself feel whatever wants to come up. Stay with it and keep breathing. As with everything, this too shall pass.

5. Replace the old habit. If you have followed the steps this far, you will realize there is a void where there was once the addictive behavior. What took up so much time and energy is suddenly gone, and a void of sorts is left. If you don't fill up that space with new and healthier practices or nurturing resources, you run the risk of falling back on your default system of acting out. Old habits are hard enough to break, but if there is nothing waiting to take their place, it's all too easy to slip into the unwanted patterns again.

Especially in the beginning stages of breaking an addiction, it is essential to have places to go and healthy people to be with. One of the best fellowship programs around is Alcoholics Anonymous or any of its sister programs like Debtors Anonymous or Sex and Love Addicts Anonymous. You can do what they call a "ninety in ninety" which means you go to ninety meetings in ninety days. For the hour or hour and a half that you sit in the room with other people who are going through similar challenges as you, you find support and inspiration. You put yourself into a safe haven where it's okay to share your feelings and concerns in the spirit of experiencing a healthy and serene life. You are reminded of where you need to take responsibility, how to make amends, when to forgive, and how to let go.

When Joe was going through his first few months of sobriety, he looked at those meetings as one would look at a cold glass of lemonade on a hot day in the desert. He would sit and listen to the other members describe their "experience, strength, and hope" until it started sinking in, replacing that old hopelessness with a new and fresh outlook on life. He looked around the room at all the people who had had similar experiences, some more rife with drama, others less so. And he became convinced that if they could get through these difficult challenges, he could too. He would come out of the meetings with slogans that kept him on track and insights that furthered his understanding of how addiction could be healed. A particularly helpful thing for Joe was that he always went to the 6:30 PM meeting, which was his usual cocktail hour, so that when his body clock alarmed him that it was time to hit the bottle, he instead shared his anxiety with his peers, thus forming a new and healthier pattern of coping.

Again, I strongly recommend the twelve-step program and other fellowship support groups. There is no replacement for the kind of wisdom and fellowship you will find in those rooms. But in addition to attending regular group meetings, there are all kinds of nourishing, life-giving experiences that can help to fill the time that the old addictive habits used to take up. For starters:

- **prayer and meditation**
- **nature walks**
- **journaling**
- **gardening**
- **a good book or movie**
- **church, temple, or any other house of worship**
- **breathing exercises**
- **dancing, singing, or any kind of artwork**
- **study with a spiritual teacher or mentor**
- **going on a study retreat**
- **talking with a friend over coffee or tea**
- **playing with or walking an animal companion**

Doing any of these things (and you can certainly find many more) will fill you up and help you to feel grounded and supported. Trust me, I know that when you are in pain and longing for the old fix, these suggestions may look like thin replacements. When I removed myself from a highly addictive relationship, gardening was the last thing on my mind. But it helped pass the time and it made me feel like I was doing something solid and healthy. That, and doing a hundred other little things helped the days go by as I built up my strength in order not to return to my drug of choice. These activities work; they help you to feel connected to yourself and the world around you.

The trick is to engage in whatever you are doing with as much full attention as you can muster. Rather than reflecting on the past or plotting out your future, try staying in the moment and experience the gifts if even for a minute or two. In this way, you will retrain yourself, consciously and subconsciously, to lean into health rather than devolve into old negative habituations.

You would also be wise to support yourself with healthy food and exercise. You can shift your focus from what used to be a ritual of getting high to a ritual of preparing a fresh organic meal for your friends. Since so much of addiction is also physiological, I include several books in the Suggested Reading section at the back of the book, any of which can guide you to eating in such a way that the cravings for the old substance or behavior will be less intense. The less sugar and refined foods you eat, for instance, the smoother your return to homeostasis (the set point of feeling okay in your body). Exercising regularly, especially out in the fresh air, will shake off nervous energy and get the endorphins flowing. By filling your day with activities that support your wellness in each of the areas of body, mind, and spirit, you will one day wake up to notice how vastly your life has changed for the better. Looking to an addiction for relief is just a maladaptive way of getting your needs met. By instead turning to trustworthy people and health-building ways of living, you will connect in a real and lasting way to the real source of happiness and peace. As you continue to work on yourself—through therapeutic means and spiritual practice—you will shift in both subtle and dramatic ways. You will find yourself attracted to different sorts of relationships and experiences while enjoying a more joyful outlook on life.

6. **Make yourself useful.** This one is more important than I can say. It is the spiritual practice that supports the physical and emotional healing from addiction. When you extend yourself for someone else, you get a better sense of how far you have come as a developing human being. You solidify your thoughts and ideas by sharing them with another person who is a few steps behind you in

their particular area of struggle. You will hear yourself speak and realize that you are wiser than you knew, and, hopefully, more compassionate than you were before starting this whole process of recovery. You will notice how much the changes you've been working on have actually set in as you lend your time and attention to someone who is still in the thick of their dark night.

There is no more estimable act than assisting someone in his or her journey from darkness to light. Your heart swells, you feel useful and worthwhile, and you forget about your own problems for a while. The self-centered fear—which is a result of forgetting your connectedness to Spirit—will dissolve as you become more present to someone else's plight. This is not the old model of being codependent, in which you forgo taking care of yourself in order to get kudos from someone you want to please; rather, you're trying on a more magnanimous version of yourself, an upgraded and more advanced evolution of who you are.

When Joe was going through his early stages of recovery, he would spend his Saturdays at a home for kids who had been abused and neglected. Because he came from the same sort of upbringing, he knew how desperately they needed to have some "safe" time with adults. He chose to mentor one child he really connected with, reading him books and teaching him how to throw a basketball. He kept patiently showing up every weekend and was thrilled to see how the boy seemed to lighten up a bit each time. The boy soon started to laugh more easily and even allowed himself to be silly (something many abused kids cannot do). Joe began to realize that his life had purpose, that he had something to give that was meaningful and unique. Later in the week when he was tempted to get into his cycle of self-pity and gloom, he would think of his mentee and his mood would lift. It was as if this service he was doing for someone else was actually medicine for his own soul. It improved his outlook on his problems (when compared with the boy's not having a home or parents, his seemed vastly more workable), elevated his sense of personal importance, and made him feel like a healer rather than a victim.

If ever you begin to feel inferior, reach out and help someone who needs it; this spirit of volunteerism will show you *experientially* that you are worthwhile and your life has meaning. Put in some time doing "the real work," and suddenly the worldly concerns, such as making money or getting ahead—all the things that made you anxious—come into perspective. As you become the person you are meant to be—kind, connected, and compassionate—you will leave behind the anxiety, the feelings of isolation and insecurity.

7. **Reinvigorate your path of healing.** In order to stay sober and keep moving forward on your continuum of health and well-being, it is essential that you keep checking in to gauge where you are thriving and to address where you are going astray. Even if you are no longer in the throes of your addiction, you still run the risk—as we all do—of falling into some old emotional traps (feeling sorry for yourself or getting overwhelmed with life, for instance). By taking a regular inventory of your feelings and actions, you can step back and do the necessary work yet again. You can ask yourself, "Where am I being obsessive and what do I need to do to get out of this rut?" or "Did I handle today's meeting conscientiously or was I acting arrogantly out of fear?"

By continuously examining yourself, you will keep clearing away the glitches in your character. This daily practice of checking out where you feel stuck or how you need to upgrade your behavior will also remind you to take care of yourself and your life in ways that might have slipped your mind. You might see that you need a few more minutes to meditate and connect with Spirit if you are feeling out of sorts or insecure. You might find that a good workout at the gym helps calm your anxieties. You might go over the day in your mind and reflect on how you were unkind to your partner, and then make amends. Or you may notice some pent-up emotional turmoil that needs to be processed by a good bout of screaming into a pillow so that you can let go of the anxious feeling you've been carrying around. On the path of sobriety we must constantly be engaged in the balancing act of surrendering and being proactive.

Life doesn't just suddenly stop being a challenge when you stop using or cease acting out on an addiction; there will always be issues and irritations to contend with. If you don't want to fall back into self-defeating behaviors, you must remain on top of your process, looking at life with what Zen Buddhists refer to as "beginner's mind," curious to see what you can learn and how you can do better.

Having someone to check in with regularly gives us objective assistance in pushing through denial and maintaining forward momentum. As we share our concerns with an open heart, we inevitably find guidance and inspiration. There is always more to learn and a deeper level to break through to; this need not be regarded as a burdensome assignment, but rather an exciting discovery of our own power and serenity.

Even when you think you are doing well, I would encourage you to run through these steps (or whatever personal process of recovery you choose to follow), because with each level of your personal unfolding, something new will occur to you. As the lessons sink in, you will go deeper and feel clearer and build an even stronger foundation for happiness.

8. Watch out for the little ones. As you master your more obvious addictions, smaller, less obvious ones might show up. You might find yourself watching too much TV or becoming attached to a certain food or overly dependent on a particular relationship. All these little obsessions and compulsions deprive us of our life force and freedom. These too can be addressed through the process described above.

Anytime you can call yourself out on being "attached" to something, it's a good idea to address it. I work with a woman, for instance, who is a successful publishing professional. She often comes home exhausted at the end of the day, her brain drained from a lot of mental work. After she puts her kids to bed, she usually "zones out" by going online and shopping for treats for her family, and she can easily get herself into a frenzy, convinced that she "needs" a new set of dishes or an area rug or coatrack and she needs it now! She knows this kind of attachment is a subtle addiction, an attachment to a rather meaningless outcome (the new *thing* that will soothe her soul). It's not a dangerous behavior; she doesn't even have a lick of debt; but it's a distraction from real downtime, and it never really gives her the relief or release she is looking for.

As I see it, it's a process of constant pruning. The healthier you become, the more clearly you can see how your energy has gotten stuck and figure out how to move through it.

Breaking free from any kind of bondage is essential. When we are wrapped up in something that takes all our attention, we cannot pay attention to the bigger issues at hand.

We are not here on this earth to indulge our every whim; we are here to become richer and deeper souls, and then push our light out into the world. In order to step up into our larger role, we must tend first to whatever holds us back.

The Circle Widens

Throughout this book we have been looking at all the means you can use to feel the very best you can. My hope is that you are learning better ways to take care of yourself so that you are happy and healthy, but also that through that endeavor of healing—of working through whatever ails or hurts you or holds you back—you become more grounded and connected and spiritually attuned so that everyone around you also benefits from your well-being.

If, for instance, you come to the conclusion that holding on to grudges has had a deleterious effect on your health, you benefit personally by attending to your lesson of forgiveness, but so does the person you were embattled with, as he or she experiences a release in his or her sense of well-being. If you decide to quit smoking, your children are also direct beneficiaries. If you decide that eating meat is no longer the right choice for you, your discovery is beneficial for you and even better for the animals who are spared. This is the ripple effect, and it's one of the most beautiful parts of this process. As we heal ourselves, others are healed right alongside us.

As we learn to take care of ourselves on every level—tend to our wounds, upgrade our habits, and lift ourselves into a higher consciousness—we free up our energy, our life force—to contribute more to the healing of the world. This is the true essence, the teaching, of healing; it is intimate, authentic, and purposeful in the grandest of ways. When you connect with your own inner physician, the remedies you discover don't only help to heal the disease or injury you are dealing with; they also redirect your energy so that you become a healer in the world. This is how we can bring about a massive shift in planetary well-being: one person at a time awakens, and with that awakening, they affect others around them. And so goes the collective awakening. The healing that started with just one person becomes an exponential—a quantum—move toward peace and happiness. One person does indeed make a difference.

Nobody knows you better than you do, so if you just take the time to be quiet and go within, the solutions to whatever ails you will appear. Whether your concerns are metaphysical, medical, or emotional, the divine physician will lead you to your cure. As it is said, within every problem already lies the solution. You need only ask yourself the questions and remain open and willing for the guidance that is sure to come.

There is more to illness and crisis than just malfunction or decay; there are stories the soul wants us to tell, lessons our higher Self wants us to embody. When we are willing to investigate the nature of our choices—how we have led our lives thus far, what our values are and how we adhere to them—we can begin to decipher the clues as to how and why we are suffering. As we step back and begin to see the bigger picture, we can respond in a truly multidimensional way, tending to body and mind and spirit at once.

Whenever you feel less than 100 percent magnificently well, say a little prayer asking for insight and guidance, then ask yourself one or more of the following questions. The answers will lead you into your healing on whatever level is necessary.

1. Where am I out of balance?
2. What am I doing that is probably harmful to my health?
3. Is there anything I am doing that is not in synch with my spiritual knowingness?
4. What do I need to learn and embody?
5. Is there a teaching that I am resisting?

6. How could I better attune myself to the healing process?
7. Is there some outstanding conflict that needs my attention?
8. What do I need to let go of?
9. Are there voices or sentiments within me that are trying to be heard? If so, what are they saying?
10. Do I want to heal?
11. What am I getting out of this current situation?
12. What can I do in the context of this situation to more fully embrace the love that is within and all around me?

If you can, take one question a day—or even a week—and meditate on it. Walk around thinking about it, talk to your most intimate friends or family about it, and ruminate on all the possible angles. There is no right or wrong answer, only insight. If you see that there are things you need to work on, map out your intentions and plans so that your path becomes clear to you. And as difficult as it may seem, allow for the idea that perhaps this illness, this being out of balance, this addiction or depression or anxiety or sadness, was a gift. Touch on the gratitude as it opens your heart.

Each of us is capable of true and lasting healing. If we are seriously ill, we must, of course, explore the rational track of medical decision; we can research, learn, and become expert on what ails us. We can seek out the best doctors, herbalists, nutritionists, and body workers possible. We can upgrade our diet, eliminate toxins more efficiently, reduce our stress, and move our bodies. And we should. But we can also ask that we be brought swiftly and gently to whatever insight is necessary in order to transcend this struggle. We can cozy up to the deepest part of ourselves and listen, making peace with all the disparate parts. Most of all, we can request a miracle. It might sound something like this:

A Prayer for Healing

I call forth all the forces of love and healing, that I might
experience a radical shift in my healing process.
I ask that this healing begin immediately.
I am ready to be cleansed and purified, and brought
up to my highest level of well-being.
I do not know what this miracle will look like, and I release
the need to oversee each and every detail.
But here and now, I make myself available to the awakening.
May my awakening lift up the whole world. And so it is.

Try this:

1. The next time you feel tempted to use your drug of choice, be it a substance or a behavior, try out a twelve-step meeting or engage in some other healthy sort of support fellowship.

2. When you are not feeling well in any area, ask yourself some leading questions that will guide you into some powerful insight.

3. Say a prayer asking that your awakening be forthcoming.

PART FIVE

Making the Leap

CHAPTER TWELVE

Be the Change
Stepping Up to the Life That Is Calling You

Be the change you want to see in the world.

—MAHATMA GANDHI

I have a cause. We need those don't we? Otherwise the darkness and the cold gets in and everything starts to ache. My soul has a purpose, it is to love; if I do not fulfill my heart's vocation, I suffer.

—ST. THOMAS AQUINAS

If there is to be peace in the world, the nations must live in peace. If there is to be peace among nations, the cities must not rise up against each other. If there is to be peace in the cities, neighbors must understand each other. If there is to be peace among neighbors, there must be harmony in the home. If there is to be peace in the home, we must each find our own heart.

—LAO TSU

WE HAVE COVERED A LOT OF GROUND IN THIS BOOK, AND IF YOU HAVE been trying the practices I've described, you are no doubt already experiencing some changes in how you feel, how you take care of yourself, how you see your "problems," how you perceive and engage with the world around you. There is one more aspect—the final frontier, so to speak—to lifting ourselves into our full potential, and that has to do with discovering our purpose. What are we doing here, after all, and what were *you* brought here to do?

As I see it, each one of us has the unspoken assignment to propel ourselves—and with us, the world—into a better place. We can do this in any number of ways, small and grand. This core purpose, when we embrace it, lifts us to feeling wonderfully alive and fulfilled. We sense that we are at last doing what we are supposed to be doing with our unique talents and position in life. Everything seems to make way for us as we rise to meet our calling: doors open, ideas start flowing, and Providence seems to usher us swiftly down this glorious path. We realize that our whole lives have brought us to this exact spot so that we can be healers. Of ourselves and of our world. We have been supported in our personal unfolding by a force that continues to bring us closer to the love within us so that we can use that love to build bridges and close gaps. This is how we weave together a brighter reality for all.

Upgrading Unhealthy Traditions

As children, we adopted our values and attitudes and ways of seeing the world from parents, teachers, clergy, and peers. Many of these templates are still with us in what I would refer to as an unconscious tradition. We didn't choose them, we simply took them on. Of course, just because we didn't choose them consciously doesn't necessarily mean they are no good! Some traditions serve our higher calling in that they bolster us with a sense of identity and strength; they provide roots in which we can stay centered even as we branch out.

Take for instance the tradition of a Native American sweat lodge: a young adult will feel ushered into maturity when invited into this ritual. He will feel that he is part of a long line of ancestors who have gained wisdom from being part of a healing and purifying practice.

This is a positive tradition, one that helps to mark growth and give comfort or inspiration. This kind of tradition is a recognized event or habit that is passed on *consciously* from person to person, generation to generation.

Of less service to you and your happiness are the negative traditions that have been passed on *unconsciously*, those that exist without examination or a higher purpose in mind. For example, we know that domestic violence passes through family lines; it is an ugly, painful, and violent tradition, passed on without awareness or any higher purpose. A boy-child who witnesses his mother being beaten by his father is statistically 30 percent more likely to beat his own wife; a girl-child who witnesses this violence toward her mother is 30 percent more likely to end up being beaten by her partner.

The point is, we are drawn into traditions—both positive and negative, by careful education or blind emulation—and it's time to discern whether they serve us or not.

I was recently looking at a house with a real estate agent and noticed that in nearly every room there was a large fur blanket made up of a collage of many different pelts sewn together and dyed unnaturally bright colors. These blankets were tossed over the beds, sofas, and even folded into the dog's sleeping area. I said to the woman who was showing me around, "How sad that so many animals had to die a miserable death so this person could have all these silly and unnecessary blankets all over her home." And she answered, "Darling, that tradition of using animals to beautify our lives has been going on for thousands of years. It's the way of the world." She was right. It was indeed a time-honored tradition, passed down through many generations and throughout many different cultures. But I wonder if she might see the wisdom in discarding that tradition, in seeing the unkindness in it and saying "No thanks."

You may have done a fair amount of soul-searching in your life.

Perhaps you've gotten some good therapy or participated in any number of self-help programs. Even so, you may be surprised to discover some of the long-held traditions that are keeping you somehow less than magnificent. If you want to excel, to be truly happy and healthy on all levels of body, mind, and spirit, everything must be brought up for assessment so that your most empowered life can emerge.

Begin by looking meticulously at your history and becoming aware of where you might be tied to old ways of being or thinking that no longer serve your evolution. When I asked a client of mine, Regina, who was struggling in her marriage to do this, she realized that she was carrying on a long-held family tradition, passed from mother to daughter, of staying with a husband out of a fear that she couldn't make it on her own. Regina, like her mother and her grandmother, married a man who "saved" her from financial worries and the anxiety that she would not be able to take care of herself. Her husband was a good man, but there was no soulful connection, only a sense of owing him a great debt for rescuing her. As we talked about the similarities in dynamic of the three generations, Regina began to see where she was locked into a holding pattern that started long before she was born. She felt, though, that she had a lot to lose by tampering with the (thus far unconscious) tradition.

All kinds of fears swirled around that tempted her to turn away from the challenge of breaking free and making a life for herself. But Regina ultimately realized that she no longer wanted to be enslaved by fear; she wanted to find her power and see how far she could go with it. She didn't leave her husband right away; in fact, it took her two years of just sitting with the realization of how and why she had landed in this place. This observation gradually led her to the conviction that if she wanted to evolve, she had to challenge herself. Regina is divorced now, and doing quite well on her own. Her career has taken a few unexpected and fortuitous turns and, although the separation was heartrending, she knows she did the right thing.

As with all the previous steps in this book, the very acknowledgment of the issue, the unconscious tradition, is enough to get the ball rolling. Remember, you can give this process as much time as you need. You don't have to make a move right away. All you have to do is recognize what you are doing. After that, the choice is yours to continue doing it or not. Just let it rise into consciousness and you will eventually access the power to change it.

Whether the tradition is a career choice (you come from a long line of doctors and are therefore expected to be a doctor even though you'd rather be painting) or personal habit (your family is a stoic one; none of you show emotions), the choice is yours whether or not to continue. The question you must ask yourself is this: *Do I want my life to be run by these unconsciously accumulated traditions, or do I want my life to be run by me?*

Carrying on unexamined traditions is what I call "living by rote." Perpetuating habits of our lineage, habits that are patterned or imprinted into us usually in childhood, is precisely how we keep ourselves—and the world—from changing and evolving. When we live by rote, we repeat the mistakes of our parents—and their parents—over and over. We sleepwalk through our opportunities, and before we know it, life has passed us by and we feel that there is something we didn't do, didn't quite rise to.

In essence, if you are living by rote, reenacting traditions you picked up from others, you aren't living your own life. You are living the life of those who had gone before you, as they lived the lives of those who had gone before them. Living by rote means not looking at what you really want, who you really are, how you truly feel, or what you truly believe in. It is doing and living without authentic thought, feeling, or clarity, and it's a sure recipe for a life of quiet desperation.

On the other hand, to live on purpose (rather than by accident) means that you consciously choose and create your life. You decide what is meaningful to you and devote your energy to manifesting it. The sense of fulfillment you can create for yourself is immense, and the good that you can do for the world as a result is massive.

Setting Your Personal and Worldly Aims

A life lived on purpose has two layers to it: on one level is your aim for personal happiness and abundance (personal aim), and on the other level is your aim for how you would like to affect the world (worldly aim). Again, this process is all about leaning into, aiming for, your most-realized potential. The first concerns getting in touch with what would help you to feel happy, satisfied, and fulfilled. I, for example, realized that I am happiest if I don't have a time schedule that I have to stick to for my work. I like to wake up with the sunrise and go about my day without rushing or answering to anyone. I also like lots of time alone so that I can process my thoughts and ideas creatively, sometimes talking out loud or daydreaming until things line up for me in my mind.

In a past stage of my life, I lived very much the opposite way. Eons ago, I used to model, so if I had a booking, I would usually wake up before dawn, rush out of the house without breakfast to get to the shoot and catch the early light. The photographer and creative director dictated the day's schedule and we models simply stood in as they created their ideas for the picture.

I knew that the career was a sought-after one and that I should have been happy with it, but I wasn't. I felt awkward and out of my skin. I always worried about not being pretty or cool enough and I felt I wasn't really contributing anything of my true nature. Don't get me wrong, for other women, modeling might be a reflection of their true nature, their art; they might be great performers or lovers of design. I was neither. Besides, I was a klutz when it came to moving and performing like the other, more talented gals did. I was living by rote, because the popular culture had told me I *should* be working to further my success as a model. I just happened to be tall enough with the right bone structure to fit the bill, but I didn't really feel like trying to strike the right attitude or dress in the fashion of the moment.

By staying with that career, I was living by rote; I wasn't living in such a way that I felt I was really contributing something from an authentic place inside me. What preceded my decision to leave that career was my realization that I wanted to live in a more purposeful way. I couldn't just stop right away because I needed the money and I didn't yet know what else I could do to make a living. So I just sat with the observation and set my intention to make a move when the time and opportunity seemed right. I started visualizing myself sleeping until I awoke comfortably, starting my day without hurrying out, and being creative and productive in the ensuing hours. When my writing and counseling career began to take off, I felt like I was living on purpose at last.

This is not to say that there were no sacrifices or compromises: I didn't have children, because they would have deserved more attention and patience than I could have given; I do have people to answer to (publishers, agents, and hosts of speaking engagements, for example), and I don't make quite as much money as a working model or commercial actress does. But all this is far outweighed by the joy I feel at being so connected to my purpose. I am happy in ways I could never have imagined.

So what about you? Consider the following questions in a way that puts you on track for rising to meet your personal aims.

1. Is there an unconscious tradition that I am carrying out? If so, name and describe it (or them).

2. If I were to live closer to my true nature, what might it look like?

3. What steps or sacrifices might I have to make, and am I willing to make them?

As with most of the questions I ask you to consider, these are designed to redirect your mental and emotional energy and move you toward a shift. Don't be surprised—and certainly don't beat yourself up—if you discover that there's a gulf between your aim and your present reality. You might well meet some internal resistance; that's okay. Simply having the questions in mind will generate a shift within you, a wave for you to ride as you reposition yourself for a breakthrough. Sit with the realizations you come up with, without pressuring yourself to do anything immediately. Rather, remain willing to answer the call when it becomes loud enough—for, surely, it will.

How Can You Be the Change?

Okay, now, how do you discover your worldly aim—something you would like to see unfold on a larger scale, be it in your town, your state, the country, the world? How do you align your "authentic self" with the great needs of the world?

The wellness of our world depends on your contribution. I don't say that to lay a burden at your feet but rather to remind you of the depth and breadth of your power. You make a difference. What you do, or don't do, makes a difference.

We are in a place and time in history when change is critical. There is so much suffering—war, poverty, cruelty, and toxicity—that if it is not addressed by more than the few who have already dedicated their lives to being activists, we will not survive as a civilization. There is more potential now than ever to cause great and grave harm: our weapons are more destructive, the appetite for consumption and profit is more callous, and a sense of injustice has fired up the desire for retribution in too many hearts. There is darkness in our world that cannot be ignored. Our light is needed. By healing our own personal lives, we free ourselves up for the larger task of healing the world.

If you don't know already what calls to you for help, turn on the news or read the paper (or browse the Internet) and really open your heart to what you hear. It might be third-world refugees, the unethical use of animals, abuse of children, environmental exploitation, or political dishonesty. Whatever agitates you the most, whatever feels crushing or breaks your heart, that is where you are called to step in.

There is no gain by trying to pacify your anger, sadness, or aggravation by turning away: common tactics to soothe frustration include shopping, obsession with tabloid fodder, watching silly TV shows, or engaging in anything that results in isolating you from the truth of what is. We are a world that is largely asleep. And as Dr. Martin Luther King, Jr., famously said, "One of the great liabilities of history is that all too many people fail to remain awake through great periods of social change. But today our very survival depends on our ability to stay awake, to adjust to new ideas, to remain vigilant and face the challenge of change."

It's not easy to let the pain of the world into your heart; it seems like a slippery slope once you start looking around and gauging how serious things are. But what if that refugee or mangled body or frightened soul were you? Wouldn't you want people to do something to help? You would indeed. I am suggesting that you turn *toward* that which is stirring you up, just like you did with your personal issues. Go into it, and be the change you wish you to see. This is how you rise to your worldly aim. Here again are a few questions you can ask yourself:

1. What makes me the angriest or saddest in the world?
2. What could I do about it that would not force others to adopt my views (whether by harassment, propaganda, or money)? In other words, how could I lovingly and compassionately help others in a way that is free of fanaticism or narrowness?
3. What are my available resources? Time? Money? Brainpower? Am I willing to give them in the service of fulfilling my worldly purpose?

Notice how you feel as you rise to the Healer within. Keep planting the seeds of peace, joy, and healing so that you continue to lend yourself to the work of transformation in the world. It is stunning how good it makes you feel, how rich and full your life becomes.

Discovering Your Authentic Nature

As we seek to discover who we are and what we are here for, there are some very positive traditions we can look to for inspiration. For instance, various native cultures use some form of vision quest to help people at turning points find and feel the truest aspects of their authentic nature. The specific rituals differ, but the essence remains the same: in order to do deep, focused work on himself, the vision seeker goes out into a natural setting alone (or with a trusted guide) for a period of time—a few hours, a day, several days, or even several weeks—leaving behind family, friends, work, and home. You can find a beautiful clearing in a national park to sit in, or pitch a tent, or stay in a small cabin that is far away from everything. In nature, we are more prone to experience the kind of gentle revelation that can coax us forward in life. We can sift through the various aspects of ourselves and come to terms with what to let go of, at the same time becoming clear on the direction of our future.

When you are immersed in the untamed energy of being outdoors, with no cars or homes or city sounds, you can better sense your own connection to that universal life force that flows through everything. Your life may be teeming with demands: mortgages and taxes, illness, work pressures, marital stress, loneliness. Whatever it is that is capturing your energy and attention, the vision quest allows you to step away from it all—for a prescribed period of time—in the spirit of reorganizing your life into a higher order. When you do that, things have a way of falling into place.

To do a vision quest yourself, find a place that is as untouched by modernity as possible. Go out into the woods or mountains or sit on a desolate stretch of beach. Commit to spending a few hours of quiet and then you can do more as you become comfortable. As you enter this natural setting, leave your issues at the periphery of your awareness. Don't try to suppress them; just place them to the side for now. Shift your focus away from trying to control or figure out how things should be and open your heart to the guidance from your inner voice.

Regardless of your dilemmas of the day, simply listen to the song of a bird. Smell the rain if it hangs in the air. Watch the sky moving above you. In this way, the guidance will make itself known to you. By shifting your attention in this subtle way, you will find a greater clarity that just seems to arise out of nowhere, and the solutions to problems will very likely become apparent to you. Once you begin to anchor your awareness in the magical beauty of nature, the next step is to listen for the messages that are sure to appear. Know that this is psychologically sound: what you're really doing is turning to the natural subjectivity of your subconscious mind, which catches at the things that will register what you need to know. As you listen to the rustling leaves, what do you hear? Seeing animals go about their business, what do you learn? What is being brought to your attention? Remember: not everything is a sign; you don't need to worry that every little sound or sight or smell is trying to tell you something. But if there is a charged feeling about something you see or hear or taste or smell, if something seems to click or jump out at you, notice what is trying to make itself known to you. Know that something in this experience is your inner wisdom being reflected back to you so that you can absorb it more viscerally.

The gift of the vision quest is the discovery that all the answers and guidance you need are available to you all the time. The key is to connect with the Oneness of which we are all a part. When you see how everything works together in nature, you realize that there is a benevolent underlying flow to things that we can latch on to and ride if we choose. In nature, there is no judgment, no ego at work. It is a perfect place in which to discover (or project) your own subjective inner knowings. Simply be present for these knowings; they will appear all around you once you are quiet enough to notice them. The next phase of the vision quest involves telling (and perhaps hearing for the first time) your story from beginning to end. It is up to you how you want to do this: you can journal or sit down on a rock and talk to no one in particular as you review the history that has brought you to where you are in this moment. Try telling your story as honestly and objectively as you can. This isn't an autobiography, but rather an exercise in bringing you around to a deeper and more resonant truth of who you are and where you are going.

Ask yourself these questions more than just once:

- *Who am I really?*
- *What am I all about?*
- *What do I need to understand?*

Then move on to:

- *Why am I here?*
- *What do I have to offer?*
- *What do I want to do?*

A vision quest is not a once-in-a-lifetime event. You can take a brief one whenever you feel the need to get some deep clarity about your life. In fact, the more often you're able to go into nature and rediscover yourself, the better. Amazingly, you will find that every time you take that time for yourself and put yourself through the questions, your experience of yourself will be different. This is a wonderful sign that you are growing and evolving. You will find stories that you're ready to complete and leave behind, aspects of yourself that have died, aspects that have been newly born, and adventures that you're ready to begin.

By entering into the quiet magic of nature, you lend yourself to the process of being cleansed and renewed, thus energizing yourself to move forward as a truer, more empowered version of yourself.

Exercise: Your Vision Quest

1. **Choose your location in nature. If you live in the countryside, perhaps you have a favorite spot that you feel especially connected to. If you live in a more urban or suburban environment, consider planning a day trip to a less-populated area; the peace that you will experience is worth the travel time.**

2. **As you enter into your chosen place, experience your senses as completely as you can. Notice the sounds, scents, and visuals. Listen with every particle of your being.**

3. **As you experience the world around you, be open for signs and metaphors that may speak to you personally.**

4. Now tell your story. You can write, talk, or even sing it. I do not recommend simply thinking about it, however. Internalizing your story could lead to almost endless contemplation. You want to somehow get it out through outward expression.

5. Begin your self-inquiry. Ask yourself: Who am I? Who am I really? Keep in mind that this is an exercise aimed at uncovering your true essence.

6. Move on to questions of your purpose: Why am I here? What is my life's mission? What do I need to do to get on track or to move more surely in the direction of my highest potential? Don't push for answers; just gently raise the questions and then rest into the awareness of your surroundings.

7. Listen to what comes up, without judgment. Remain open and receptive to your own inner voice and to what you notice around you. Be willing to carry this new knowledge back out into your world so that you can act on it appropriately.

Find out what makes you tick—both in the personal and worldly arena—and become the person you would be if you were doing and being everything to fulfill your potential. This is your life's work.

Keep doing the exercises in this chapter and you will come to a deeper and deeper understanding of yourself and your true calling in this world. If you've tried them just once, you have no doubt discovered many new things about yourself and touched places in your heart that were previously concealed by false beliefs and unhealthful traditions subconsciously picked up from parents, peers, and other outside influences. You are more focused on who you are and why you are here at this particular time in history; you have a greater sense of how you are to "be" in relation to the world. You have new goals, visions, and aspirations that will serve not only *your* sense of wellness, but also the well-being of the world.

Now it is time to begin ushering these new goals and visions into reality. Once you've taken a close look at the false beliefs you might be dragging around with you, decide that you're ready to let go of everything that isn't essentially, truly you. Put yourself on a schedule if that feels right to you; do things in a way that is comfortable and sensible, and in a loving manner. In other words, you need not walk out of your job or marriage tomorrow. Rather, begin to act in ways that move you closer to your goals in a way that is integral and kind to everyone involved. By doing this, you will feel lighter; you will have a sense of yourself as being on track and moving swiftly along your continuum of conscious evolution and wellness. With this newfound lightness, you might want to add some new beliefs and affirmations, some "thought seeds," to your bag of tricks that will help bring your goals and visions into reality. Here are a few examples:

1. I see the magnificence of who I am and what my purpose is; I am manifesting great things because of this.
2. I am committed to happiness and peace.
3. Abundance is mine when I live in a truthful way.
4. All of the good I want for myself I also want for everyone else.
5. As I lift myself up, I uplift my community and the world.
6. I have rich resources within and all around me.
7. I have access to unlimited willpower, endurance, and focus within myself.
8. I am connected to Spirit, and am therefore capable of anything.

9. **Everything that I do adds to the momentum of healing and wellness.**

10. **I embody the perfect balance of surrender and action.**

These are just a few examples of new ideas. You can plant and begin to integrate these ideas into your own belief system. Invent some of your own and practice giving them expression.

Honoring the Fellowship of All Beings

At times in your life you may have convinced yourself that you could go it alone, that you didn't need anyone or anything in particular to complete you. Bravo! Especially for women, this can be a huge step. But the fact is, we do need to feel connected—to ourselves and to each other—in order to thrive in a world of six and a half billion people. If we don't cooperate in a culture that is so overlapped and interconnected, we run the risk of feeling tossed out of the creative engine that makes things go round and round.

Yes, it is important to embrace our individuality and look out for ourselves; that's how we get ahead and feel a sense of accomplishment and pride. But just as a single cancer cell breaks away from the rest of the healthy cells to do its own thing, we create ultimate havoc by not considering and working toward the health of the whole—the whole of our body, mind, and spirit as well as the whole of all life everywhere.

We are all—on levels seen and unseen—interrelated. I may specialize in one thing that you need, and you can provide something else that I need. And consciously or unconsciously, we seek each other out to work through the wounds or unenlightened places within so that we can become ever more whole and happy. None of us exists or works in isolation, and it benefits us to find a way to function together in a finely tuned balance for the well-being of the individual as well as to maintain a healthy life everywhere for all.

This means we have to consider how to best take care of ourselves while also caring for the world we live in. If we fall short, the world is diminished in some way. If the world goes down, we go down with it. This requires that we look several steps behind to examine the process by which things have arisen and several steps ahead to see how our choices play out; and it means that we have to consider others as equally important to ourselves. If you think of yourself as an arm (or finger or hip) in the body of humanity, you know that it doesn't matter how much you take care of that arm if other places in the body are not cared for. If the overall body (including the heart, skin, liver, and lungs) are neglected or abused, the body will break down and very probably speed toward death. Simple as that. The arm will not, in due course, thrive if the body does not thrive.

Interestingly enough, medical science has now proved that we are healthier when we are socially aware. We are, in fact, genetically predisposed to need one another. Like bees, ants, wolves, penguins, dolphins, gorillas, lions, chimps, orcas, and other species, we humans are social by nature. We function at a higher level and with better health when we have fellowship. In fact, historically speaking, our survival has always been dependent on social support. The evidence of countless studies demonstrates this fundamental truth. For example, of 1,500 people followed for ten years in Australia, the Centre for Aging Studies revealed that those who had the fewest friends were outlived by those with a network of friends by 22 percent. Enjoying camaraderie is not only good for your emotional well-being, but also for your health. As reported in the *Journal for Cancer*, women with ovarian cancer with ample support from friends had lower levels of IL-6, a protein associated with more aggressive cancers.

Women with weak support systems had 70 percent higher levels of this same cancer-enhancing protein, and it was two and a half times more concentrated directly surrounding the tumor(s).

At Rush University, in Chicago, researchers found that seniors who feel lonely are more likely to develop Alzheimer's-like dementia. There's even a type of dwarfism that is psychosocial and has been observed in abused and neglected children. Psychogenic dwarfism is a growth disorder that occurs in children between the ages of two and fifteen in which cognitive abilities degenerate, and growth stops, regardless of the volume of food that is consumed, as long as the child is in isolation. Growth hormone secretion decreases, resulting in short stature, a low weight that is inappropriate for height, and immature skeletal age. As soon as the child is removed from isolation and stress and perceives a loving environment, physical growth and cognitive abilities resume. In addition, studies have also shown that after suffering a heart attack, a person with friends tends to live longer. And even though being around a lot of people may expose you to more viruses and bacteria, it has been proved that socialization is more potent at preventing illnesses than is avoiding exposure to germs.

It's not just the value of being surrounded by others that these studies point to, but rather the importance of feeling connected, of not feeling lonely or isolated. You can be alone with your dog and not feel lonely. And you can be in a crowded room with "friends" or family and feel achingly cut off and alone. The essential thing is to feel known—that there is a reciprocal awareness and care for another that is real and heartfelt.

So, as we come to a close, ask yourself these questions and allow yourself to be motivated to adjust your energy so that you—and the whole of everything—benefit:

1. What do I need to change in the way I eat, work, worship, and communicate that will not only bring my energy up, but also benefit every aspect of life?
2. How can I integrate my health with the health of the whole (everyone and everything in the world)?
3. Where am I predisposed to being selfish and how can I adjust that so that I feel both fulfilled *and* conscientious?
4. Do I feel connected with other people? Do I need to expand my web of relationships?

How you choose to live now—today—will not only dictate the way your personal prospects unfold, but will also help to determine the future prospects of humankind. We are all connected by our source, each made up of the same stuff. Modern physics has proved what spiritual sages have been saying for thousands of years: that all matter is essentially vibrating energy. We consist of moving electrons, protons, and neutrons and these bare components when investigated more closely really just drill down to vibrating energy that has no boundary. Essentially, beneath what appears to be our skin and bones and cells, we are bare *beingness*, shifting and flowing energy operating under the illusion that we are separate and apart from each other.

If we choose to view the things that happen in our lives (yes, everything!) as means toward our evolution, as steps in our growth and awareness, life itself will acknowledge our commitment and open to us. In fact, we will keep evolving whether by our own volition or not. But I would much rather choose to grow than be hauled into it, wouldn't you?

The more you *lean into wellness,* the more you cultivate it—be it through conscious eating, visualization, service, or good communication—the more likely you are to reach a tipping point in your life, finding yourself "all of a sudden" delivered to a new level of being, a level of extraordinary all-around wellness. And as you move along and experience these upturns, you lift the world right up along with you. You become the Healer that this world is aching for.

Where there is illness, loneliness, or a lack of vitality, apply the salve of wisdom that you have been gifted with. Stitch together your wounds so that you can be more whole and available to gather into your arms the wounded of this world. This is your work, to heal yourself, to lift yourself up and into the next level. And as you do, we all will take that quantum leap with you—into a healthier, kinder, more loving world.

May you be well in every way right now and always. May you be the healer you were meant to be. May we all rise together into a glorious new moment of awakening. And so it is.

APPENDIX I

Vitamins and Supplements

FINALLY, A FEW WORDS ON VITAMINS AND SUPPLEMENTS. I KNOW A fair number of vegetarians who didn't eat vegetables (other than potatoes) before they went vegetarian and aren't about to start now. And that's obviously true for meat eaters too. That's why I recommend taking some nutritional supplements. I say this not because our food can't supply us with everything we need, but because most of us don't eat enough fresh fruits and vegetables (three to five servings a day are recommended by the USDA) or whole grains to satisfy all our needs every day. Of course you should try, but it can't hurt to have a little insurance.

For starters, take a **good multivitamin.** Look for a food-grown, mostly organic one; it should be either time-released or require that you take a few over the course of the day.

Vitamin C is one of the most thoroughly researched of all the vitamins. A convincing body of clinical research says it is a prime protector from damaging free radicals (which cause aging and disease), so it remains the gold standard for antioxidants. It is also highly effective in maintaining a healthy immune system. You may be familiar with the work of Linus Pauling, who suggested megadoses of this wonder vitamin, and I know there's some controversy about that, but 1,000 milligrams per day won't hurt you, and will probably help you, especially if you aren't eating copious amounts of green leafy vegetables and organic seasonal fruits. It also helps the body absorb iron.

B complex (including B-12). The B vitamins are good for the nervous and digestive systems. They are easily lost in the refining or cooking process and can be diminished by heavy sweating, or drinking a lot of alcohol, tea, or coffee.

Vegetarians often lack vitamin B-12, and there's an interesting story behind why. The common story is that vegetables just don't have B-12, but that's not necessarily true. It's a matter of how sanitized our food supply has become. B-12 is produced by micro-organisms (bacteria) that no longer make their way into vegetables that are cleansed of all "dirt." Animals, on the other hand, eat and drink a lot of dirt throughout the day, and the B-12 from the bacteria gets into their flesh and is then passed on to the carnivores who ingest them.

Supplemental **iron** is vital for many of us, especially women of childbearing age who may be anemic. Although, contrary to what you may have heard, vegetarians suffer less frequently from anemia than meat eaters do, it's still better to play it safe (again, because we may not eat the amount of vegetables that we need), especially since anemia is so common in young women, whether they eat meat or not. We need iron to make hemoglobin, which carries life-giving oxygen to the cells. Be sure not to take it with other vitamins, especially calcium, as they can cancel each other out.

Flaxseeds and flax oil are an excellent source of omega-3 fatty acids (and are also a good source of omega-6). Flaxseeds, with all their omegas, are said to be an anticancer food because of the fiber and anti-inflammatory properties. Flax is also reputed to lower bad cholesterol, boost your immunity, increase metabolic rate, and be a brain builder. It was often used to heal in the times of the Roman empire and Hippocrates (the father of medicine) apparently used it as one of his valued medicines. I love the nutty flavor of freshly ground flaxseeds (two tablespoons in a coffee grinder will do the trick). I mix them into smoothies, oatmeal, and soy yogurt. Flax oil is good to add to your diet as well (poured over hot cereal, salads, toasted bread, etc.) because you need many more omegas than can be provided by just a couple of spoonfuls of seeds. The oil tends to go rancid quickly, so be sure to buy it in small amounts and store it in a dark bottle in the refrigerator. Walnuts are another great choice for omega-3s.

Vitamin D is best absorbed by spending fifteen minutes a day in direct sunlight. It boosts your immune system and reduces the risk of many cancers, so while a lot of sun can cause cancer, a little can prevent it. If sunshine isn't available, take a supplement.

Amino acids are the building blocks of protein, and they play a critical role in our physiology. Whether you are eating meat or not, poor digestion and stress can deprive you of these essential elements. If you want to make sure you are getting everything, there are plenty of amino acid supplements available at your local health food store, or pharmacy, but your doctor should test your blood and overall health before you take anything.

Once you've made your way to a plant-based diet, you would do well also to take your efforts further by avoiding sugary drinks (including a lot of fruit juice; try squeezing half a lemon or lime into some sparkling water with a touch of agave) and snacks, eating organic foods as much as possible, using natural sweeteners that won't spike your blood sugar levels, drinking plenty of water, eating three meals per day (with healthy snacks in between), trying to focus on whole foods (i.e., not refined ones), and avoiding hydrogenated oils and other foods high in saturated fats.

It may seem like a lot to think about at first, but really, eating well is just a new habit to get into. Like everything else that we are evolving into, a healthy diet is something best approached knowing that we are on a continuum. Set your sights on integrated health, and then lean into it, taking one step at a time until you have a quantum breakthrough.

Here's to your health and happiness!

SUGGESTED READING AND VIEWING

Alcoholics Anonymous. *Daily Reflections: A Book of Reflections*. New York: Alcoholics Anonymous World Services, 1990.

Alcoholics Anonymous. *Living Sober*. Center City, MN: Hazelden, 2002.

Barnard, Neal and Bryanna Clark Grogan. *Dr. Neal Barnard's Program for Reversing Diabetes: The Scientifically Proven System for Reversing Diabetes Without Drugs*. New York: Rodale Books, 2007.

Barnard, Neal. *Food for Life: How the New Four Food Groups Can Save Your Life*. New York: Three Rivers Press, 1994.

Campbell, T. Colin and Thomas M. Campbell II. *The China Study: The Most Comprehensive Study of Nutrition Ever Conducted and the Startling Implications for Diet, Weight Loss, and Long-Term Health*. Dallas: BenBella Books, 2006.

Chödrön, Pema. *When Things Fall Apart*. Boston: Shambhala, 2005.

Esselstyn, Caldwell B. *Prevent and Reverse Heart Disease*. New York: Avery, 2007.

Lappé, Frances Moore and Anna Lappé. *Hope's Edge: The Next Diet for a Small Planet*. Los Angeles: Tarcher, 2003.

Lappé, Frances Moore. *Diet for a Small Planet*. New York: Ballantine Books, 1971.

Laszlo, Ervin. *Science and the Akashic Field: An Integral Theory of Everything*. Rochester, VT: Inner Traditions, 2007.

Mills, Milton. *The Comparative Anatomy of Eating*.

Naparstek, Belleruth. *Staying Well with Guided Imagery*. New York: Grand Central Publishing, 1995.

Newport, John F. *The Wellness-Recovery Connection: Charting Your Pathway to Optimal Health While Recovering from Alcoholism and Drug Addiction*. Deerfield Beach, FL: HCI, 2004.

Ornish, Dean. *Eat More, Weigh Less: Dr. Dean Ornish's Life Choice Program for Losing Weight Safely While Eating Abundantly*, rev. ed. New York: HarperCollins, 2001.

Oz, Mehmet. *You: The Smart Patient: An Insider's Handbook for Getting the Best Treatment*. New York: Free Press, 2006.

Pert, Candace B. *Molecules of Emotion: The Science Behind Mind-Body Medicine*. New York: Simon & Schuster, 1999.

Pert, Candace B. and Nancy Marriott. *Everything You Need to Know to Feel Go(o)d*. Carlsbad, CA: Hay House, 2007.

Petralli, Genita. *Alcoholism: The Cause and The Cure*. Santa Cruz, CA: Alternative Approaches to End Alcohol Abuse, 2007.

Robbins, John. *Healthy at 100: The Scientifically Proven Secrets of the World's Healthiest and Longest-Lived Peoples*. New York: Random House, 2006.

Robbins, John. *The Food Revolution: How Your Diet Can Help Save Your Life and Our World*. Boston: Conari Press, 2001.

Sarno, John E. *The Divided Mind: The Epidemic of Mindbody Disorders*. New York: Harper Paperbacks, 2007.

Scully, Matthew. *Dominion: The Power of Man, the Suffering of Animals, and the Call to Mercy*. New York: St. Martin's Griffin, 2003.

Tuttle, Will. *World Peace Diet: Eating for Spiritual Health and Social Harmony*. Brooklyn, NY: Lantern Books, 2005.

Weil, Andrew. *Spontaneous Healing : How to Discover and Embrace Your Body's Natural Ability to Maintain and Heal Itself*. New York: Ballantine Books, 2000.

Wilber, Ken. *Grace and Grit: Spirituality and Healing in the Life and Death of Treya Killam Wilber*. Boston: Shambhala, 2001.

Films on Animal Issues

Foer, Jonathan Safran. *If This Is Kosher*, documentary short, 30 minutes. United States: PETA, 2004.

Monson, Shaun. *Earthlings*, documentary, 95 minutes. United States: Shaun Monson, 2003.

Robbins, John. *Diet for a New America*, documentary/drama, 60 minutes. United States: Community Television of Southern California, 1991.

Schonfeld, Victor. *The Animals Film*, documentary/drama, 136 minutes. United Kingdom: Beyond the Frame Ltd., 1981.

Thomas, Antony. *To Love or Kill: Man vs. Animal*, documentary/drama, 60 minutes. United Kingdom: HBO, 1996.

Websites for All Things Animal and Vegetarian:

http://farmsanctuary.org
http://humanesociety.org
http://www.meat.org/
http://peta.org
http://vegcooking.com/
http://www.vegsource.com/

Green Sites:

http://earth911.org/
http://www.thedailygreen.com/
http://www.aboutmyplanet.com/
http://www.nrdc.org/

Addiction Recovery Websites:

Alcoholics Anonymous: *http://www.alcoholics-anonymous.org*
Adult Children of Alcoholics: *http://www.adultchildren.org/*
Al-Anon/Alateen: *http://www.al-anon.alateen.org/*
Emotions Anonymous: *http://www.emotionsanonymous.org/*
Overeaters Anonymous: *http://www.oa.org*
Sex Addicts Anonymous: *http://saa-recovery.org/*

To Find an Integrative Doctor:

http://www.integrativemedicine.arizona.edu
    Click on "find a graduate"

Other Books and CDs by Kathy Freston:

http://www.KathyFreston.com

INDEX